WA
THE ART OF BALANCE

KAKI OKUMURA

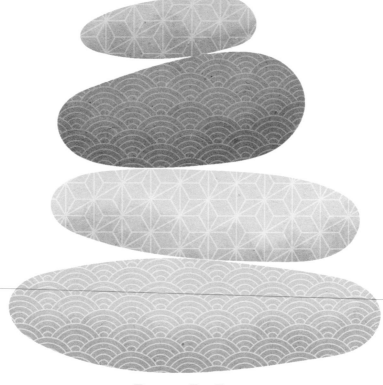

WA
THE ART OF BALANCE
LIVE HEALTHIER, HAPPIER AND LONGER
THE JAPANESE WAY

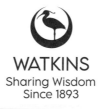

WATKINS
Sharing Wisdom
Since 1893

WA – The Art of Balance
Kaki Okumura

First published in the UK and USA in 2023 by
Watkins, an imprint of Watkins Media Limited
Unit 11, Shepperton House, 83–93 Shepperton Road
London N1 3DF

enquiries@watkinspublishing.com

Commissioning Editor: Ella Chappell
Assistant Editor: Brittany Willis
Head of Design: Karen Smith
Interior Designer: Kieryn Tyler
Cover Designer: Alice Claire Coleman
Production: Uzma Taj

A CIP record for this book is available from the British Library

ISBN: 978-1-78678-689-0 (Hardback)
ISBN: 978-1-78678-690-6 (eBook)

10 9 8 7 6 5 4 3 2 1

Printed in China

www.watkinspublishing.com

CONTENTS

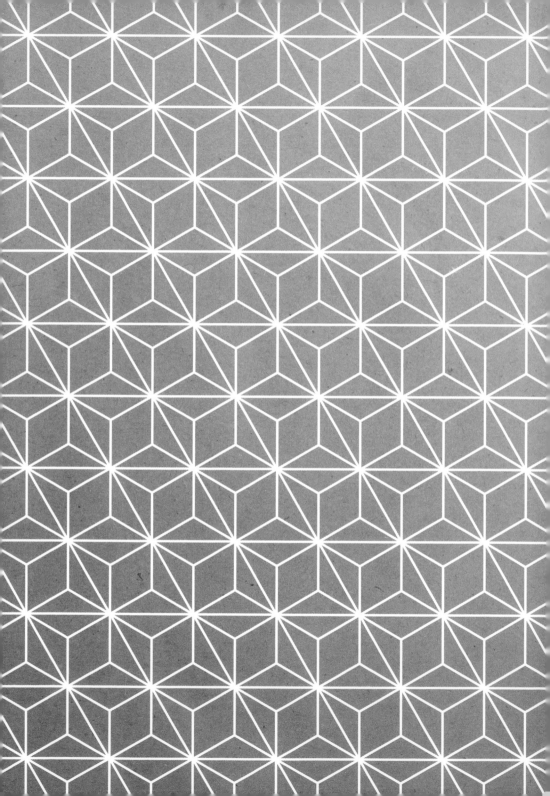

INTRODUCTION:
WHAT YOU WILL GAIN FROM THIS BOOK

How can we live healthfully? It's a seemingly simple question with a simple answer, but it's a question that many of us have struggled with. On the surface, most people will give you the generic answer: eat plenty of fresh fruits and vegetables, and exercise regularly. This is not new information, and while we recognize it as timeless and true, it's hardly helpful because it doesn't recognize people as complete and nuanced individuals. When it comes to health, we can't just follow the math – we also need to be empathetic about what makes us human.

An approach to our health that is empathetic of our humanness is not just the easier way, it is also an approach that is much more successful than one that is driven by forceful willpower. For our health is not just something we can invest in for one month, six months, or a full year and then forget – it is something that we need to be able to sustain for the rest of our lives. Day in and day out, we engage with our health every day.

It's curious because when we think about the meaning we want to derive from our own life, many of us spend a lot of time thinking about our careers. We ask questions like, what is my dream job? What kind of career and position will grant me freedom and fulfillment? How can I find this while still making a living that can sustain my lifestyle? We consider our values, our hobbies, our favorite luxuries, and our family.

"We can clock out of a job, but we can't clock out of our health."

We ask these questions because we understand that we will spend almost half of our waking life working and so we might as well find something we enjoy, rather than suffer through the first job that crosses our path. We see that salary is not the only thing we should consider, but we think about our working style, culture fit, and how our career will impact not just the bottom line but multiple facets of our life. A dream job at one point in our life is not a dream job at another, and so we also see the value in revisiting these questions and checking in with what will truly make our life fulfilling.

Yet as a society, we tend to forget to afford this same level of consideration to our health. We don't ask the same questions or revisit them with the same frequency and level of reflection as we do our career, but our health is just as impactful, if not more. Our physical and mental health affects every facet of our life – we can clock out of a job, but we can't clock out of our health.

Like an unfulfilling job, a way of taking care of our health that is driven by willpower will eventually burn us out and make us want to quit. But a lifestyle that is intentional, one that is directed by our values and joys, is one that we can and will want to sustain for the rest of our lives. It means being able to enjoy cake to celebrate birthdays, eat local foods when we travel, spend time with our friends, and do whatever it is that brings us fulfillment and meaning in this life, without having to worry about our health all of the time. Sustainable health is a way of living that makes us feel confident, joyful, and spirited. We deserve at least that, and so let's afford the same level of intention to this crucial aspect of our lives.

Understanding how to take care of my health is not something that has always come naturally to me. I was overweight as a child, and carried that identity with me throughout my formative and most vulnerable years. When we're young, an idea of health that is purely directed by looks or weight can be an especially difficult narrative to shake.

It may be helpful to share a bit about myself: I am Japanese but was born in the United States and spent my childhood years growing up in Dallas and New York, and because of this, I was raised with American sensibilities when it came to health. I saw things as "go big or go home", and that to embark on a healthy lifestyle change was one that necessitated an extreme makeover or to completely change my life somehow. I saw it as a process that required grit, perseverance, and hard work. I measured it in terms of the number of calories I consumed and burned, and the number on the scale at the end of the week.

At one point I felt like I had tried everything within my power, and because I was easily impressionable and desperate to change, I had pushed myself to go to extreme lengths and ended up on the other end of the spectrum in weight – but still found myself just as unhappy and stressed about my health. Would taking care of my health always have to feel so difficult?

This perspective changed when I moved to Japan. I saw and experienced how people did not see health as a list of things they should or shouldn't do, but that living healthily was a balancing act. It didn't require extreme intervention or change, and most importantly I was able to find an approach that aligned my health with my values – it was a way of living healthfully that wasn't governed by restriction or willpower but was rather rooted in freedom and intuition.

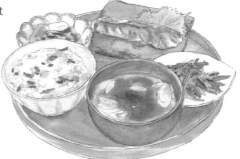

In this book I won't lecture on the importance of eating vegetables or regularly moving your body, and how it is good for our health and wellbeing. I will instead assume that these are recognized truths and offer a way to incorporate it into our modern lifestyle in a way that anybody can adopt. No matter where you are in your health goals, whether this is your first or twentieth attempt to approach your health differently, the advice is meant to be adaptable to any lifestyle, at any age, to any person. I hope you find it surprisingly effortless.

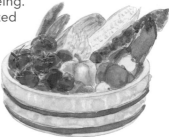

In an approach that puts human empathy at the forefront is the implied understanding that our health and wellbeing is not just our physical health but is also closely related to our mental health. In fact, these two components work in both directions – when we take care of our physical health we find that our mental health benefits, and when we take care of our mental health we find that our physical health also improves. The reverse can also be true, that when we are in poor physical shape our mental health struggles, and that when our mental health is not great, our physical health can also suffer. They're so closely interrelated that we cannot think about one without considering the other.

This acknowledgement means expanding our understanding of health beyond just eating vegetables and exercising. Many factors affect our wellbeing, and I have learned to frame our health through four essential pillars:

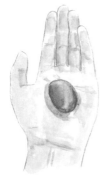

1. Nourish
2. Move
3. Rest
4. Socialize

It does not necessarily mean that Nourish and Move represent our physical health, and that Rest and Socialize represent our mental health – for each pillar there is a consideration to both. For example, eating well is not just eating vegetables; it is also important to our health to make room for foods that are celebratory or bring us comfort. Or having a robust social life is not just something that can boost our sense of belonging and confidence, but is also something that can make a marked difference on our physical health.

These pillars are also closely interrelated with each other: when we have good-quality sleep, we have enough energy the next morning to move and exercise our bodies. When we spend the day actively socializing with our loved ones, we are able to fall asleep much easier at night. When we eat well, we have the energy to be active during the day. When we're active during the day, we sleep well at night. In both obvious and nuanced ways the four pillars are all connected - what strengthens one pillar can strengthen another; overdoing one pillar may cause you to neglect another. No pillar is more important than the other, rather it's a network of support and balance.

This is *wa* (和) or the art of balance. *Wa* is colloquially recognized as a character to describe Japanese things - *washi* is Japanese paper, *washoku* is Japanese food, *wafuku* is Japanese traditional clothing - but its meaning was derived from the idea of harmony, the simultaneous combination of different factors in our life that together can create a beautiful sum. In this way, when I describe how to live healthier the Japanese way, it is less about a "Japanese" lifestyle but is about principles that are rooted in a lot of Japanese culture and tradition: the belief that to live well is to live in balance.

At the end of the day, a healthy lifestyle is not about eating vegetables or getting enough exercise, but it's about investing in a lifestyle that allows us to live out our most meaningful and fulfilling lives. It's a sustainable mindset that allows us to do the things we love with the people we love, in a way that empowers and inspires us daily: it promotes independence, freedom, and strength, but is also mindful of empathy, curiosity, and joy. We can embody these values and find true lifelong health when we discover a lifestyle balance with our four pillars.

So let's begin!

PILLAR 1:

NOURISH

It seems that everyone has an opinion on what is the best way to eat. It's been ingrained in us since we were schoolchildren that healthy eating looks a certain way – plenty of vegetables, fresh fruits, whole grains, and lean proteins. This is not technically wrong, but this messaging also demonized "unhealthy" foods. Healthy eating looked like it was only vegetables, fresh fruits, whole grains, and lean proteins; everything else was essentially equated with poison.

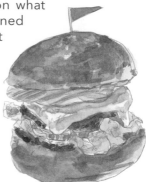

"Cut out sugar!"

"Fat is bad!"

"No more carbohydrates!"

"Eliminate dairy!"

Even without those formal structures of school or healthcare, advertisements and online presences send – overtly or covertly – messages as to what it is that we should be eating every day. Children today are probably receiving many more messages than generations earlier as media becomes more ingrained into our everyday lives.

Even as an adult, it is a difficult landscape to navigate. One year it seems that we should all be avoiding saturated fats, and the next year we are told that carbohydrates are the enemy. Or is it sugar now? Most recently it seems that not only are macronutrients being criticized, but even the time at which we eat. Yet with all of this advancement of research and supposed innovation we have not solved the problem of eating well, and by certain measures, global health is getting worse.

The ironic and confusing thing is that while we are being lectured as to why sugary desserts or fat-heavy meats are bad for our health, we have culturally put them at the center of our celebrations and commemorations. We eat birthday cake on birthdays, eat burgers and fries at sports games, or go out for steaks and ice cream when we get a job promotion. Modern culture has made us believe we need to simultaneously self-restrict the exact foods we emotionally tie to positive occasions. And this "food on a pedestal" mindset coupled with a stress of what to eat or not eat has made many of us feel out of control with food.

But food shouldn't be, and doesn't need to be, a source of stress in our lives. What it should really be is an element of our lifestyle that brings us health, fulfillment, and vitality, which means to also recognize it as not just fuel, but as something that shapes our culture, identity, and joy. In this way, I feel as though understanding the art of eating as "nourishment", or sustenance necessary for growth, healing, and good physical and mental health, is the most accurate way we can think about it.

The following lessons are designed to help one adopt and understand how to eat for nourishment, a practice that is mindful of our humanness. Rather than telling you which vegetables to eat and explaining why they're good for you, I'll be sharing with you the overarching concepts and principles of balanced eating instead, so you have a timeless practice of healthy eating that is adaptable to your lifestyle at any point in your life. You'll never have to worry about how to eat well again.

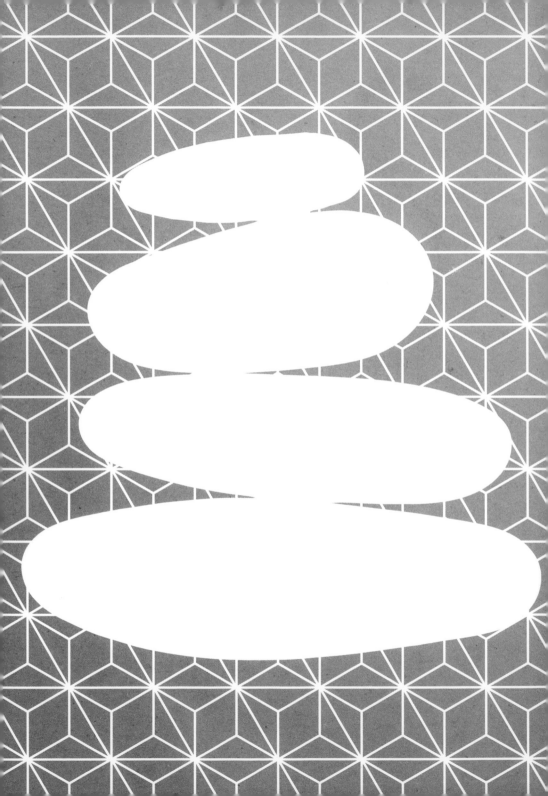

LESSON 1:
STICK WITH SIMPLE

Does everyone think about calories as much as I do?

When we think about eating healthier, one of the first strategies we undertake is calorie counting. Multinational companies such as Weight Watchers or MyFitnessPal have made large fortunes from this simple idea: Eat fewer calories than you burn, and you will lose weight and be healthier. Under-500 calorie meals and 100-calorie snack packs are popular marketing techniques, and often when we look at a nutrition label it is the largest text on there. We think of it as one of the most important – if not the most important – factor to pay attention to in our food.

Yet the healthiest foods available to us don't come with nutrition labels telling us how many calories they contain, so if you were to eat healthfully you'd have to go to a lot of effort to track every single calorie you were consuming. How many calories are in a head of broccoli? A bowl of spinach? A cup of strawberries? The majority of people don't know, and hundreds of millions of people have lived perfectly long and healthy lives without ever knowing.

We don't need to calorie count to live a healthy life, but does this mean that we shouldn't? It depends on who you ask, and this is where reflecting on our personal values can help.

What kind of lifestyle would allow you to live the most meaningful and fulfilling version of your life? It may be helpful to take a moment to think about how you like to spend your free time, who you like to spend it with, and how tracking the minutiae of your food intake makes you feel. Can counting calories factor into that vision?

I cannot speak for everyone's experience or values, but the majority of us, even if we were to successfully reach a certain weight through counting calories, will think that this strategy is not aligned with our values. It can make us obsessed, distrustful of our bodies, and constantly worried about "watching our weight" even when we are within a perfectly healthy range. Counting calories for weight loss works from a purely scientific sense, but human health is not just physical – our health encompasses our internal sense of contentment and wellbeing.

There is a way of addressing healthy eating without having to even think about calories. In fact, sometimes the less we think about such things, the healthier we can become physically and emotionally.

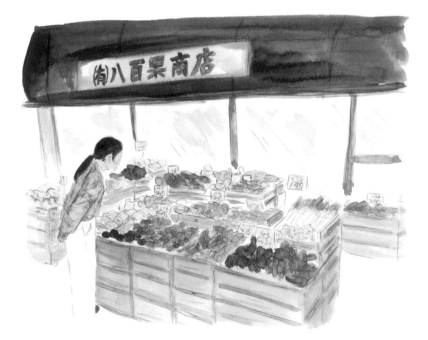

It was a strange summer in Tokyo when I discovered that.

Our memories are in many ways inaccurate, but one thing they are really good at telling us is what we were paying attention to at the time. We remember the big, emotional events, the things that can impact us and linger in our mind afterwards. And what do I remember when I think about that summer in Tokyo? It wasn't calories. I have no idea how many calories I was eating. But I remember two things clearly:

1. That I was eating a lot of delicious food. Mochi cakes, ice cream, matcha shaved ice, sushi, yakitori, fried noodles, and fried chicken wings, just to name a few. It was a joyous time.
2. It was also the first time in my life that I was able to successfully lose some of my excess weight.

I didn't even realize I had lost weight until my mother pointed it out to me. I decided to step on the scale to disprove her beliefs, and the sheer shock of seeing a lower number after a summer of eating without concern left me wondering for months afterwards: What had happened? Was I inadvertently eating some miracle fat-burning Japanese superfood? Or was simply eating without thinking the golden rule I'd been missing?

Turns out, it was none of the above. Returning to the US, I quickly gained back whatever weight I had lost, and then some. It took several years after that summer for me to really understand what had happened and how I could be conscious of it, rather than hoping for the sheer blind luck of it to manifest itself again. But it came up in my mind again and again: If we don't need to pay attention to calories when it comes to our diet, what do we need to pay attention to?

I made it my mission to find out.

In my pursuit of the answer, I came to realize I had naturally become a healthier weight during my time in Tokyo because I was doing daily things differently that summer; I just didn't recognize it at the time, for it was neither remarkable nor particularly revolutionary. It was simple.

When habits and mindsets are simple enough, they become intuitive, and the practice of taking care of our health can feel as natural as brushing our teeth in the morning or combing our hair. We don't see these things as critical to our health because we don't really think about the importance of, say, brushing our teeth, but go a few days without it and you'll quickly see how the small things add up when it comes to our wellbeing.

If we had to pay attention to the amount of toothpaste we use, or the brand of toothbrush we are using, or at what time we have to brush our teeth every night, the complexity would be exhausting. The sheer thought of taking care of our dental hygiene would make us want to give up. But luckily, we don't need to expend our energy like this to have healthy teeth, and the same idea can apply to eating.

We don't need to put in lots of thought or energy following a complicated meal plan or dogmatic diet to live healthfully. In fact, if we keep the practice simple, we can make it as natural as brushing our teeth before going to bed or combing out our hair before we leave the house in the morning. It is in this mindset where true sustainability and long-term wellbeing can finally take place.

So that is lesson one.

Lesson 1: Stick with simple

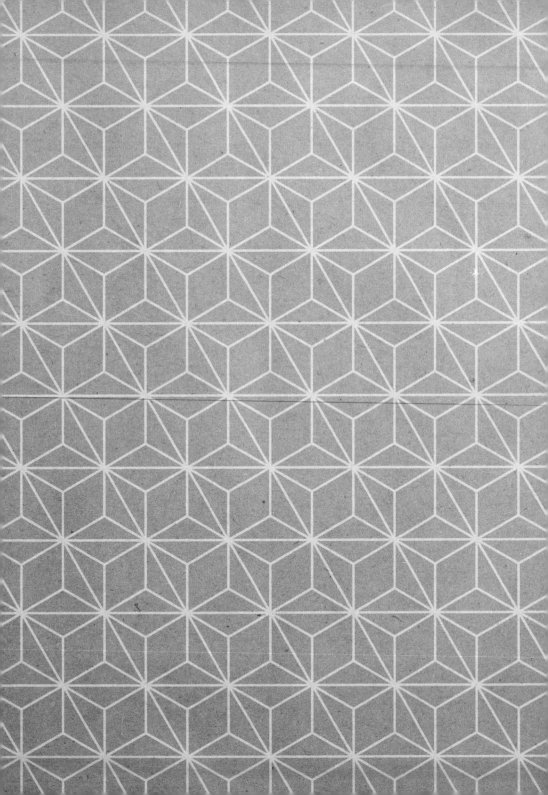

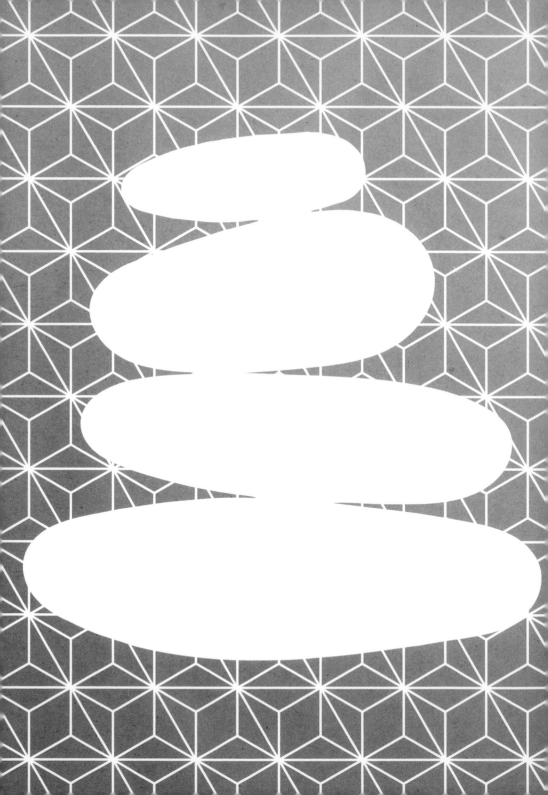

LESSON 2:
DESIGN FOR
HARAHACHI-BUNME

"Itadakimasu!"

The first night back in Tokyo was always my favorite. My grandmother would welcome us into her home with ready-made futon beds, a gigantic order of sushi waiting for us on the dining room table, and a selection of fancy Japanese *wagashi* confectionery sweets sitting in the fridge for later.

She didn't serve us any grocery store-type sushi either, but a large round platter freshly delivered from the sushi restaurant one block over, where the vinegar rice was at the perfect temperature, and the fish was unfailingly tender and generously served.

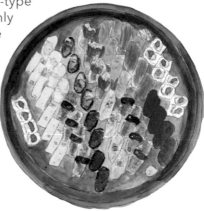

But there was always something very unfortunate about this first night back in Tokyo that made this homecoming meal a bit of a struggle: I was never hungry for it.

This was quite reasonable because the time difference from New York to Tokyo is 13 hours in the summer, meaning that a 6pm dinner time in Japan actually feels like a 5am New York morning to someone who has just arrived. Not to mention the 12-hour flight during which you are sitting and doing nothing, so it is no wonder that I never felt hungry.

But I love sushi, and I especially love the sushi from that restaurant, so it was always my inclination to eat a lot even if I was not hungry. It is hard to describe why my need to eat felt so strong even when I had no appetite – was it the anticipation? The emotional attachment to the event? That I had not had this sushi for so long and didn't want this moment to slip away? While I had never really confessed out loud how I was never hungry for this first meal back, my grandmother was a perceptive woman, and she would see that I was forcing myself to eat.

"*Harahachi-bunme, Kaki-chan.* Don't worry about having to eat everything right now. You will probably feel hungry when you inevitably wake up in the middle of the night, and there will be plenty left waiting in the fridge for you."

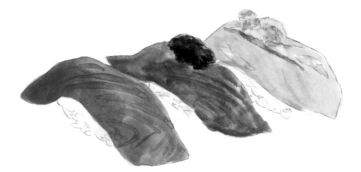

Harahachi-bunme directly translates to "80 per cent of your stomach", or the idea that we don't need to be eating until we are full, only until we are satisfied. At 80 per cent, we feel neither overstuffed nor deprived, but satiated and content. The phrase is actually part of a longer Japanese proverb, "*Harahachi-bunme, isha irazu*", which translates to "Eat in moderation, and you will never need to see another doctor."

When my grandmother said this to me, I didn't give her words much consideration, but I realized later that it was an idea that ended up sticking with me, whether I was conscious of it or not. *Harahachi-bunme* is not just something my grandmother adheres to; the concept is omnipresent throughout Japanese society, and so even without thinking too hard about it I would find myself being nudged toward moderation.

For example, have you ever seen those videos online of "How is McDonald's in Japan Different?" or "What Do They Serve at a Starbucks in Japan?" If you watch one of these videos, you will often find that the host will order and review the different kinds of food and drink offerings, such as Teriyaki Burgers, Ebi Filet-O, and Roasted Green Tea Frappés.

But they consistently miss the most important and notable difference between a McDonald's in Japan versus the United States, a difference that almost always comes up in conversation whenever I talk to someone who has visited Japan, whether they be an expat who has spent many years living there or just a tourist strolling by.

"If they tried to pull the same stunt in the United States, there would literally be riots."

"Then again, the United States can probably learn something from Japan."

"It would explain why Japanese people have a much easier time staying lean."

What are we talking about? Portion sizes.

Food sizes are surprisingly arbitrary and inconsistent, even within the same brand. I used to be shocked when I would go to a Japanese McDonald's. When I ordered a medium-size beverage I would think that it was almost childishly small. "How could anyone consider this cup to be an acceptable size for an adult?" I'd wonder. The ironic thing was that coming back to the US after a few months, I'd again find myself thinking, "How could anyone consider this cup to be an acceptable size for an adult?" Only this time, I'd be astounded by how big a medium-size beverage in the US is: a medium in the US is 21oz but a large in Japan is 20oz. How could a US "medium" size be larger than the Japanese "large"!

It's not just McDonald's – this phenomenon is present in fast food chains and restaurants across the board. I remember visiting a Starbucks in NYC and ordering an iced latte, only to remember after I paid that I forgot to tell them that I wanted the size "Tall". The cashier didn't ask me, but I assumed that I would be charged the Tall size anyways, as in my mind it was the most typical size. But when they called my name, it was in a Venti cup – which is double the size of a Tall! It was the difference between 12oz and 24oz; his default idea of a typical drink size was much bigger than mine.

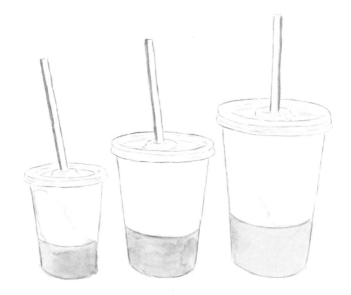

I could've just brushed this off as a one-time event, but when I went home to look it up, it turns out that the perception of a proper drink size is actually quite different between the two countries. Did you know that the most popular drink sizes at Starbucks are different in Japan versus the US? I hypothesize that it actually has nothing to do with personal preference, but because of the way the menus are designed.

To explain: Starbucks in Japan has a "Short" size (8oz) listed on its menu – the menu display shows sizes Short, Tall, Grande, and sometimes Venti. Consequently, because there is a size Short on the menu, the most popular cup size in Japan is a Tall, because it's considered the middle size. But if you wanted to get a cup in the size "Short" in the US, you'd have to make a special request for it, as it is not written anywhere – the menu displays only Tall, Grande, Venti – and consequently, the most popular cup size in the US is a Grande because of the "middle option bias" or the tendency for people to choose the moderate option when presented with three competing choices.

A small French fries from Burger King Japan is about 75g, whereas a small French fries from Burger King US will be almost double that at about 130g.[1] As of 2022, Burger King UK doesn't even offer small fries anymore, and the smallest size available begins at 116g. The smallest Domino's pizza in Japan comes in a size "M", a 9-inch diameter (22.9cm), whereas the smallest size, "small" in the US, is 10 inches (25.4cm). There are many examples of how the default sizes can vary immensely between different countries.

This is how I've come to realize that subjective labels are prevalent throughout the food industry – a medium in one context is not necessarily a medium in another. Labels such as small, medium, and large are relative, and so when considering our own diet it is important to be mindful of the default portion sizes that are being offered to us rather than accepting them without regard. We should be mindful of checking in with ourselves: how much do I actually want to eat?

The concern of relying on default sizes extends to not just fast-food places, but to eating out at typical restaurants as well. If you visit a restaurant in Japan, the meals are portioned so you're expected to comfortably finish it in one sitting, and so taking home leftover food is a very rare and uncommon service offered at restaurants. If you asked for a takeout box, your server would probably look at you with a very strange face!

Yet eating out in the United States, restaurant meals are often impossible to finish without a takeaway container at the end. Asking for one is normal and quite often expected, as the portions served are purposely very generous - a nice benefit if you're attentive to your fullness, but the caveat is that if you are not exercising mindfulness, you can quickly overeat.

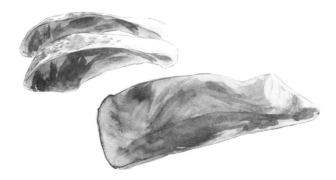

The difference between default food sizes is also pervasive in our grocery shopping environment. Take, for example, the case of buying salmon fillets: in Japan, if you buy a single fillet of pre-cut salmon it will probably weigh about 80-90g. This is standard, and if you wished to buy a fillet of a bigger size you would have to visit a specialty fishmonger counter to create the slice for you. In comparison, visiting a grocery store in the UK, you will find that it's about 120g. In the United States, a single fillet is often sold as a little less than half a pound, or about 200g. That's more than double the size of a Japanese fillet!

Of course, you may argue that you could simply slice the salmon fillet in half yourself, but if you didn't know or look up what the recommended serving size for salmon was - the Harvard T.H. Chan School of Public Health says it's about 3oz, or 85g - and then compare that amount to the weight printed on your grocery, then you could end up eating double the recommended amount without ever knowing. It's an extra step that most people just don't have the time or inclination to always engage with.

A common myth in the world of health is that the more willpower and effort we expend, the higher the rate of success with our health goals. We've been told that if we just exercise self-control, command discipline, follow a diet, and become stricter with ourselves then the process is easy – but my time in Japan has shown me the exact opposite. It's not about personal willpower, but the little unconscious things in our environment that nudge us.

I used to refer to *harahachi-bunme* as "the Japanese rule to a healthy diet", but if you were to go up to a typical Japanese person and refer to it as a diet protocol or rule of any sort, they would probably correct you and tell you that it's not really. Instead, it is more closely considered to be a lifestyle principle that allows moderation to become the natural inclination.

Japan is consistently a country that is a leader in longevity[2] and maintains very low rates of obesity[3] – the least among high-income, developed nations at 4.3 per cent – because it has successfully managed to maintain a societal environment where default portion sizes are smaller, allowing its population to consistently eat at a moderate level, or *harahachi-bunme*, while paying little attention to the matter.

You may be thinking along the lines of, "I don't live in Japan, and I have no intention or ability to move there any time soon. I can't change my environment, so what can I do?"

I get this response frequently whenever I share insights with someone who is trying to adopt principles of moderation for themselves. But we don't need to live in Japan to do this because we don't have to eat to *harahachi-bunme* for every meal for the idea to have an impact on our health. We just need to practice moderation the majority of the time.

So first we should focus on being intentional about the space where we spend the majority of our time eating. Where is that for most people? Our home.

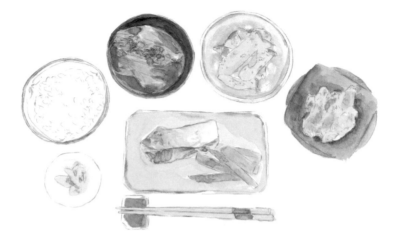

Many Japanese meals are modeled after the idea of *ichiju-sansai*, or "one soup, three sides", where small plates are combined to compose one whole meal. The one soup refers to a bowl of miso soup, and the "three sides" refers to two small vegetable dishes, and a single serving of a protein dish, most commonly fish. Served with a bowl of rice and maybe a *tsukemono* pickle topping, *ichiju-sansai* style meals are a popular way of eating at home.

When I speak about *ichiju-sansai*, I frequently receive the follow-up question, "White rice? Aren't refined carbohydrates bad for you? Won't it cause my blood sugar to spike and lead to insulin resistance?" or "Why do Japanese people stay so lean even though they eat so much white rice? That's so much sugar."

It's not a myth that Japanese people eat a lot of rice: on average, a modern, typical Japanese person consumes 82.1kg (181lbs) of rice per year[4] – for comparison, Americans consume about 10.8 kg (24lbs) per year. It's not the "healthy" kind of brown, black, or multigrain rice either: the rice that is served in Japanese school lunches, government cafeterias, and in the typical Japanese household, is plain, short-grain white rice.

The narrative around carbohydrates seems to always be changing. One year I'm told that carbohydrates should be making up the majority of my diet, and the next year I hear through popular media that in fact I should've been following a no-carb diet this whole time.

As we cycle through several dieting trends in our lives, most of us have come to believe that not all carbohydrates are bad. We admit the health benefits of fiber-rich starchy vegetables, and are less opposed to brown rice, barley, oats, and other forms of whole grains. Yet enjoying refined carbohydrates still seems wrong. It's not uncommon for people to talk about white rice or white bread as if it's a cigarette, and for it to be associated with terms like "dangerous", "cancer-causing", and even "poison". This narrative has been so pervasive in the personal health world that many of us probably know of someone who will regularly drink alcohol but resist eating white bread. There is so much fear around it.

Strong taboos against entire categories of food are not exclusive to refined carbohydrates; it is a narrative that strikes most food groups, from fat, to dairy, to sugar, to meat. Almost like gossip, popular nutrition advice – which logically should be unchanging over a lifetime – tends to shift from one year to the next, sometimes taking on a complete 180 reversal of what was being advised before. Surely not everything can be bad for your health?

A trending dialogue which feeds into fear of food is one that is always troubling to me, because fear of food does not solve our health problems, and can often exacerbate it. Even with the best intentions, for some people genuinely think that they are doing others a favor by sharing these messages, a fear of food only feeds into our anxiety, and anxiety is never an effective way to build the foundation of our wellbeing.

Some may argue that this fear is necessary in some cases, to encourage individuals to change their lifestyle habits and become proactive about their personal health. We all need a push sometimes, no? The problem with an approach rooted in fear is that it is what leads many people to extremism, whether this be undereating, overeating, stressful and time-consuming diets, or an obsessive relationship with food. It ends up impacting our self-esteem and our sense of self-control, and from this point many people end up doing even crazier and more extreme things to try and regain that control, such as avoiding eating with others, performing elaborate food rituals, and weighing out the ingredients in every meal.

At its core, a healthy lifestyle is about investing in what brings us more energy, joy, and fulfillment – but if food obsession becomes the forefront of one's lifestyle, it is no longer part of building that foundation. It is no longer healthy.

So does that mean white rice is good for you? Does that mean you can eat it endlessly and not worry about any consequences? Not necessarily, for there is an art to enjoying all kinds of food healthfully, and it comes back to moderation.

If you look at Japan where white rice is a beloved staple, a plain bowl of rice is never the entire meal: it is often served with fish, meat, soups, salads, and other vegetable dishes. One part of a colorful whole, or within *ichiju-sansai*. Moderation is about looking beyond the specific food and seeing its role on a larger scale – any kind of food consumed in excess is not good for our body; conversely, any kind of food consumed in moderation is perfectly adaptable into a healthy lifestyle.

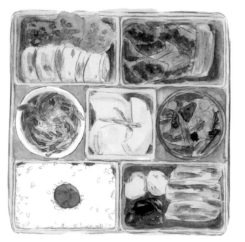

White rice is not necessarily celebrated as a healthy food in Japan, but it is not considered a dangerous or unhealthy grain, because it exists in a lifestyle where it is part of a larger balance – no stress, no obsession, no shame, and no guilt. It is just food. And when we design our meals with moderation, not extremism, in mind, we are able to regain control of our wellbeing and build a foundation toward health that is sustainable for the long haul.

Moderation is easy to talk about, but when it comes to the practice it can be intimidating for a lot of people. What does moderation actually look like? How should one approach it? Can people really trust themselves to be intuitive toward the amount they eat?

As a first step I always recommend to people, instead of becoming too hyper-focused on what moderation should look or feel like in any context, see where you can start with your plate sizes at home.

You'll notice that when enjoying an *ichiju-sansai* meal, individuals are rarely actively thinking about the amount that they are eating once they've sat down. Instead, this thinking is done beforehand, when they are plating their food: a moderate portion of miso soup, rice, vegetables, and fish onto single serving-size dishware. There's little need to think about eating in moderation, because the dishware's size helps nudge one in the right direction.

So, start with your dishware at home. It's the best place to start because it's where we eat most often, can exercise the most control, and can experiment continually as we navigate new approaches. If you don't already have single-serving dishware at home, Japanese grocery stores or online vendors often offer bowls or plates that are of single-serving size and purchasing a few to use at home can assist your own understanding of moderation.

> "A healthy lifestyle is about investing in what brings us more energy, joy, and fullfillment."

To clarify, using smaller bowls to nudge ourselves toward more moderate portions is not about restriction – it's important to give yourself permission to eat as much as you want – but when we serve ourselves a little less to begin with, we create a crucial pause for mindfulness to take place. It might not seem like much, but it's just enough space and time to ask yourself:

1. Do I feel stuffed or starved?
2. Am I thirsty or hungry?
3. How will I feel after another serving?

And by being more conscious of how we feel after finishing what's on our plate, we will begin to achieve what feels right at 80 per cent full, or *harahachi-bunme*, a balance where we are neither overeating nor depriving ourselves.

Lesson 2: Design for *harahachi-bunme*

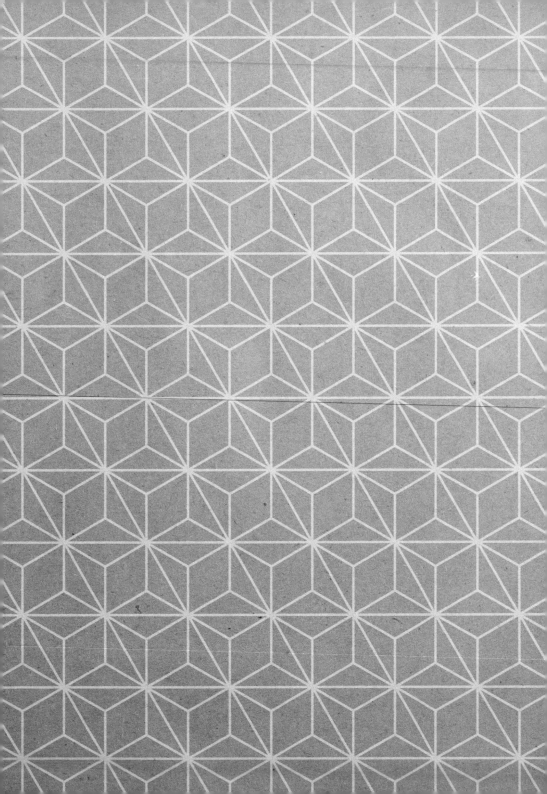

TORORO FURIKAKE RICE

(2 servings)

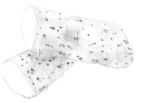

It is on almost every Japanese
teishoku restaurant's menu,
but I never ordered it because
I thought it was the oddest
thing. Grated sticky yam on
rice? Who thinks of that? But
take note because it turns out
this mountain yam will boost your rice game and
you'll never want to go back – in fact, it's not just
delicious but it's sometimes referred to as "mountain
medicine" because of the yam's natural digestion-
boosting enzymes. Serve it warm or cold, you can
enjoy this dish all year round.

Ingredients
- 1 nagaimo (also known as Chinese yam – or
  "mountain medicine" in Mandarin – it is an almost
  bewhiskered, tubular root vegetable often found
  in most Asian food stores)
- 200g/7oz cooked rice
- 1 tbsp water
- 1 tsp dashi powder
- furikake (Japanese rice seasoning) to taste

Instructions

1. Peel the nagaimo and grate it down. Add water and dashi powder, and mix together in a bowl – this is tororo!
2. In a separate bowl, mix together rice and furikake.
3. Serve the rice into single serving portions, and top with the tororo.

Note: Nagaimo or Chinese yam can be eaten raw, but other yams can't, so do not substitute a different kind of yam or potato here!

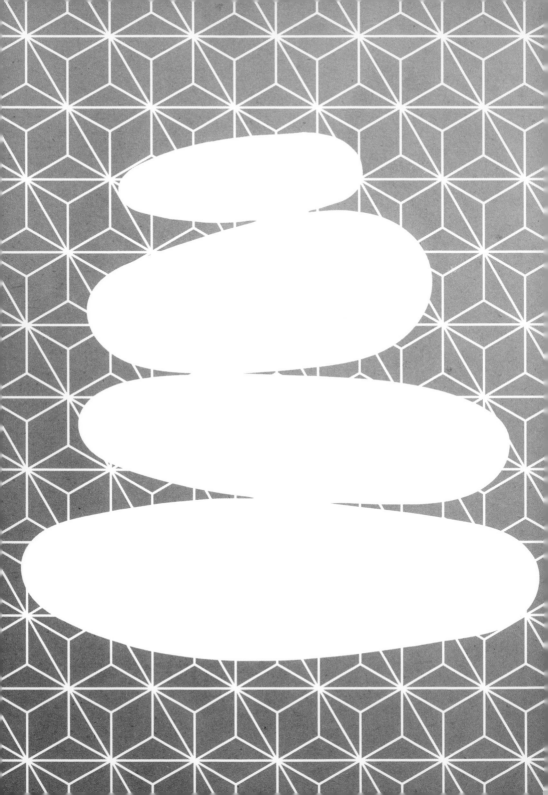

LESSON 3:
SEEK VARIETY

The key to achieving and intuitively understanding *harahachi-bunme* is eating whole, nutrient-dense food. While not strictly in the saying, 80 per cent full is best understood and realized when we are eating foods that help signal satiety and satisfaction, something that is not always possible with modern food products.

Have you ever opened a box of cereal and just found yourself unable to stop eating it? Or perhaps it was a can of Pringles, or a tray of Oreo cookies. You have probably come across an instance where you picked up a snack and found it difficult to stop eating. Calorie-wise you may have thought you'd start feeling full after a while, but somehow we find that the sense of satiation never arrives.

It seems strange that there exists food in our world that the more you eat of it, the more you end up wanting to eat, but if you pick up a typical packaged or processed snack at the grocery store, more likely than not it will make you feel this way. It's not because we are undisciplined and out-of-control individuals, it is because our natural biology cannot accurately read cues from these sorts of processed foods.

While it may not seem so anymore, cereal is a very new invention when it comes to human existence. It was popularized during the large-scale development of the "Big Food" industry around the 1950s, which centers on the creation of food products that are not conducive to satiation: hyperpalatable and appetite-increasing foods are the most profitable, so it goes without saying that manufacturers have carefully designed packaged foods to include lots of sugars and salts – and remove satiety-signaling nutrients like fiber – to be as addictive and tempting as possible.

While I don't believe in having to cut out these foods from our diet wholly – I enjoy snacks and think processed foods can be safely included in what we eat – if our diet is based primarily on processed foods, our body cannot accurately measure nourishment and hunger from these mostly "empty" or nutrient-deficient calories. It leads to overeating because these foods take us way beyond the point of fullness before we even begin to register it, making it much more difficult to sense and stop at a point of moderation.

When designing a healthy life, it is important to focus on fruits, vegetables, proteins, and whole grains, so our stomach and brain can respond accordingly to our needs. We will not only stop feeling unnecessary hunger, but we will also lose the desire to eat with abandon; eventually, preventing overindulgence will not be a test of willpower, and can feel like a natural response.

You don't have to completely eliminate snacks, desserts, or other foods that you enjoy to achieve this intuition – in fact, I often encourage individuals to create space for these foods, as strong-arming elimination can lead to obsession and guilt. Instead, what this means is that we should tastefully embed these foods in a diet that is primarily of whole and fresh foods, so you are still able to meet natural cues of satiation, while feeling confident in your intuition and the food choices you make.

So how can we balance the "healthy" with the "not so healthy"? If you're unsure of what this balance may look like, let me first pose a question for you: what do you think of when you hear "fried chicken meal"? Growing up in the US, I was very accustomed to thinking of something along the lines of a six-piece fried chicken, side of French fries and a small Coke. Even at a young age I quickly understood that fried chicken for lunch was not considered a healthy meal.

So imagine my surprise when I was with my friend in Tokyo and instead of the standard six-piece with French fries I was accustomed to seeing, her fried chicken meal came with a beautiful assortment of chilled sesame tofu, *okura natto*, *wakame* miso soup, *hijiki* rice, and daikon pickles. Yes, it was still a fried chicken meal, but it almost looked … healthy?

In retrospect it may seem like such an obvious idea, but it was at that moment I realized that fried chicken doesn't need to be served with fries and a soda.

It is not just this one meal at this particular restaurant either, where fried foods are served with a healthy variety of fiber-rich vegetables and food types. Consider the typical Japanese tonkatsu, or fried pork cutlet, meal. If you ever visit a tonkatsu restaurant in Japan – which I highly recommend; it's delicious – you may be surprised by what each of the deep-fried pork cutlets are served with. They are not served with mashed potatoes or macaroni and cheese, and never a side of fries. They are consistently served with raw shredded cabbage and a bowl of miso soup.

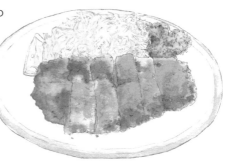

Why is that? According to Japanese legend, the now-conventional pairing was actually first a random accident: when tonkatsu was first brought into Japan during the Meiji era[5] the dish more closely resembled the schnitzel you'd find in Vienna or Germany, served with a side of potatoes and sautéed vegetables. But due to the mandatory draft for the Russo-Japanese war in 1904, one tonkatsu restaurant owner suddenly found his kitchen short of hands. To save time, he changed the menu so that the pork cutlet would be served with raw shredded cabbage, rather than cooked vegetables.

After a while, the restaurant found that the raw shredded cabbage was much more popular among diners. The customers would say how they liked that it freshened the mouth and it didn't make them feel so heavy after. The restaurant gained a lot more popularity after the switch, and other restaurants began to serve their tonkatsu with shredded cabbage. The trend persisted until today, and now Japanese pork cutlets with shredded cabbage is the classic way to serve the dish.

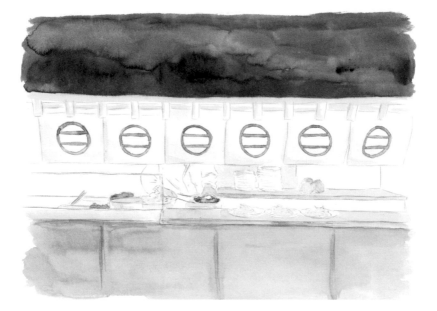

It may have been discovered by accident, but there is a very thoughtful balance taking place: the dietary fiber in cabbage[6] suppresses and slows the absorption of fat from the pork cutlet and helps feed healthy gut bacteria for digestion. Cabbage is also rich in an enzyme known as s-methylmethionine, also known as vitamin U,[7] which gently protects the gastrointestinal membrane of the stomach. This enzyme is particularly abundant in cabbage but is altered with high heat, but when consumed raw one can enjoy the full benefits of it.

"Maybe you can't change the world, but you can make it the way things are done and preferred in your own home."

Imagine if restaurants in the US began to serve all of their deep-fried dishes with miso soup or plain raw cabbage! It may seem like an impossibility, but it is culturally commonplace in Japan: like how serving burgers with fries is the convention in the United States, serving tonkatsu with shredded cabbage and miso soup is the convention in Japan.

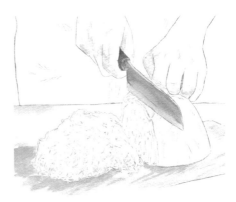

Maybe you can't change the world, but you can make it the way things are done and preferred in your own home. Consider serving your fried dishes not with buttery potatoes, but with a refreshing salad to balance, or your cheesy casserole dishes with salted, juicy tomatoes to complement. You may assume that the best way to enjoy a hefty burger is with a side of fries, but let yourself be creative!

You don't need to deviate too far from what you're familiar with to find a more well-rounded balance with your meals. For example, coleslaw is another popular side dish to burgers, but consider swapping the classic version for something that is lighter on the mayonnaise, and you may find that this version complements the dish better. Experiment a bit further, and you may even find that a side of raw shredded cabbage is the best way to enjoy it! There is no single best side dish to our meals, but I encourage you to hold an open attitude and broaden your horizons – maybe adding something contrasting and fresh to the side is what will bring your dish alive. The food pairing conventions we are used to are simply just conventions, and with a little thought and creativity, we can open ourselves up to a whole new world of deliciousness.

The traditional Japanese meal set *ichiju-sansai*, or "one soup, three sides", helps individuals accomplish this balance with little effort: rather than seeing a traditionally unhealthy food – such as fried chicken or pork cutlet – as something to be eliminated from the diet, when combined with a vegetable dish and miso soup into an *ichiju-sansai* meal, one can achieve eating healthfully with few restrictions.

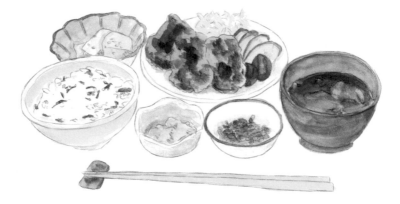

Centering our idea of healthy food around variety is not about reducing our caloric intake or lessening our intake of fats and sugar specifically, but is about making healthy eating sustainable. It allows us to engage with a thoughtful balance and reduce the risk of a common all-or-nothing breaking point, and diversity in the foods we eat also allows us to find better balance with our overall health.

The success of variety as a principle for healthy eating is not just a thought experiment: variety has shown to be one of our best tools in graceful aging and healthy living, especially when we are able to embrace variety in fresh vegetables and whole fruit.

A short trip to Okinawa showed me that.

Okinawa is an island prefecture in southern Japan that stands out among a country that is already well known for longevity. It doesn't just boast beautiful beaches, crystal-clear waters and lots of sunshine; it is famously known to be a "Blue Zone",[8] a region of the world identified to have a higher than usual number of centenarians.

So what allows them to stay so healthy? If you were to ask a Japanese person what the longest-living Okinawans eat that allows them to live so long, they might mention the vegetable goya, or bitter melon.

Goya is often colloquially known as "the Okinawan superfood" and credited for the prefecture's healthy population. It's a cucumber-shaped vegetable with bumpy dark-green skin, and, as its English name suggests, it tastes quite bitter. Okinawan home cooking is well-known for its use of this vegetable, so much so that they have a day dedicated in May to goya, and if you were to visit a souvenir shop at the Okinawan airport you would probably find a few goya-themed keychains and t-shirts. It is high in vitamins B, C, and K, and is also known to be frequently used in traditional Chinese medicine as it is believed to help blood circulation, reduce the risk of chronic diseases, and promote healthy digestion.

Does it sound too good to be true? I had the opportunity to visit Okinawa one summer, and of course I was curious to experience the wonders of goya and see how they incorporated the vegetable in their diet. It is the key superfood that allows the people of Okinawa to enjoy such a long and healthy life, after all! I was prepared to ship a box home and begin using goya in all of my meals.

"Variety has shown to be one of the best tools in graceful aging and healthy living."

It is not false that goya is just about as healthy as it sounds – the bumpy, bitter green vegetable is rich in several vitamins and is a good source of antioxidant compounds that can help protect your cells.[9] When I was visiting and dining at Okinawan establishments, I typically saw at least two to three items on the menu that used goya, most cooked into tofu stir-fries or tossed on top of salads.

But I was surprised to find out that outside these Okinawan restaurants, goya consumption was far from a daily medicinal routine, but simply another vegetable that one may enjoy. Speaking to the locals during my time there and from a quick google search on a few forums, it turns out that most people in Okinawa don't necessarily eat it that often. Not significantly more than they'd enjoy other vegetables such as carrots, spinach, or tomatoes at the very least. In fact, goya is regarded as a biting, controversial vegetable among Okinawans: some people love it, some people hate it, and while it's an Okinawan cultural icon, most people only have it on occasion. It's a typical point of view most of us have with any vegetable.

> "We don't need to learn new recipes or cooking methods to expand the variety in our meals."

But it is true that Okinawa produces significantly more centenarians by percentage than the national average in Japan, and it seems that they don't just live long, but they live healthy and active lives well into old age. A 2007 study on Japanese centenarians living in Okinawa analyzed until what age these individuals were able to live independently – defined as cooking for themselves, doing their own house chores, and living in their own home – and made a fascinating discovery: The study was only on 22 individuals, but among them, 82 per cent were still independent at a mean age of 92 years and about two thirds were independent at a mean age of 97 years.[10] In other studies it was found that among Okinawa's elderly, dementia is less prevalent[11] compared to the general population, and research from 2014 found that their heart disease or breast, prostate, and ovarian cancer is also lower. Their lives are not just long, but also remain healthy well into old age.

So if it wasn't the superfood goya, how do these individuals eat differently compared to the average person? In an interview with CNN, the researcher leading the study, Craig Willcox, shared that he found these Okinawans typically eat seven different fruits and vegetables a day, and more than 200 different foods and spices regularly in their overall diet. He credited not a single vegetable for their good health, but variety.

When I first came across this study, I was shocked at how they managed to include so many different vegetables in a day. It seemed like a lot of work, and I didn't think this approach could be conducive to the modern lifestyle – these Okinawan individuals were probably in a special environment where that was manageable, but I couldn't possibly eat like that forever. Busy people don't have the luxury of time to create such varied meals.

But if you consider one of the most common and famous Okinawan foods, a stir-fried vegetable dish called *chanpurū*, maybe this isn't so difficult. *Chanpurū* means "to mix together" and can be a variety of different vegetables, but a classic version would include goya, tofu, egg, and bean sprouts, sometimes with carrots, cabbage, or onions. This dish is often served with a side of steamed sweet potato and a bowl of miso soup, which is frequently made with seaweed, tofu, and daikon radish. Okinawans also often enjoy a portion of fruit after or between meals, such as pineapple or papaya, with some freshly brewed jasmine tea.

It's not just *chanpurū*; many Okinawan dishes are an assortment of different vegetables, such as *jūshī* or papaya *irichī*. These are dishes that aren't particularly difficult or time-intensive to make. At their core they're simple stir-fries, but these dishes are consciously constructed with many different ingredients in one dish. Suddenly I could see how incorporating many vegetables into one's day could be manageable.

Though Okinawans are famous for their good health and longevity,[12] the reason why the Okinawan diet works is not due to any vegetable found in their environment or elimination of any particular ingredient from their diet. It is because of an approach in cooking and eating that results in a lifestyle where most meals are diverse, colorful, and regularly include an assortment of leafy vegetables, root vegetables, and sea vegetables, without having to make any single ingredient the center of one's diet.

We don't need to learn new recipes or cooking methods to expand the variety in our meals. For example, if you have plans to make some soup for dinner, try throwing in some spinach or a can of crushed tomatoes that you otherwise wouldn't have added. If you're making pasta, add some color by tossing in a handful of peas or sliced mushrooms. You can add some avocado to a rice bowl, sliced fresh tomato to a sandwich, or get creative with anything else that's sitting in your fridge. It can be as simple as adding some sliced apples to your usual breakfast, or blueberries to an ice cream dessert at night – think in terms of adding to what you already enjoy, rather than reinventing your entire meal plan. Small changes add up.

The principle of variety is not just limited to fruits and vegetables but can also be applied to other food types and spices. In Japan it is popular to add a variety of different grains like millet or barley when making rice to make *zakkokumai*, for added color and texture, or red adzuki beans to make *osekihan*, for a slightly nuttier and sweeter rice.

People will also often top their rice with furikake, a Japanese seasoning that is traditionally made of dried fish (most often bonito), dried seaweed, sesame seeds, salt, and a bit of sugar. Furikake was first invented by a Japanese pharmacist named Suekichi Yoshimaru during the Taishō period (1912-1926) as a simple and accessible way to address calcium deficiency in his patients. The original version was a powdered mixture of fish bones, roasted sesame seeds, poppy seeds, and seaweed – a product he named *Gohan no Tomo*, which translates to "friend of rice" – but today there are hundreds of different rice seasonings, and most families will keep a few variations in their kitchen cabinet to season their dishes.

Shichimi or "seven tastes" is another staple Japanese seasoning blend – made up of ground red chili pepper, Japanese *sansho* pepper, black sesame seeds, dried orange peel, ground hemp, poppy seeds, and *aonori* seaweed – and also has its roots in herbal medicine. Developed in 1625 in the city of Edo (now Tokyo), it was first sold as a herbal supplement marketed for its medicinal properties and was often sold in front of temples and shrines. Eventually the spice blend spread outside of Edo and became a seasoning staple for Japanese food. Today it is often used to top off udon or soba noodles, miso soups, or rice.

Variety can also be about modifying classic recipes. For example, it is popular in Japanese baking to use okara powder, or dried soy pulp, to replace a portion of a recipe's flour requirement to add an extra boost of fiber and nutrients. It's not about replacing the entire recipe with okara powder, but just a portion of it to maintain the original recipe's flavor while still being mindful of variety. Even if we don't have okara powder available to us, we can think about variety in a similar way by choosing to use some wholewheat flour in our cookies or mixing in some nuts in our brownies.

Similarly, in Japanese cooking, tofu is used to modify meat dishes in the interest of increasing variety – not to replace meat. Living in the United States I would meet a lot of people who aren't the biggest fans of tofu, even when they want to add it into their diet. Tofu is high in protein and low in calories and fat,[13] and much more environmentally friendly than proteins like beef or chicken. But it seems that a lot of people have a hard time getting over the taste – they describe it as bland, spongy, and the rawness of the soy flavor as not very appetizing.

This confused me at first, but now it's easy to see why. Western cultures have championed tofu as the optimal protein alternative for vegans and vegetarians, something to replace meat. Especially for firm tofu, this branding makes it seem like meat's less flavorful, squishier, "healthy" alternative. Tofu teriyaki bowls and BBQ tofu stir-fries don't quite ring as appetizing as meat, and many of these recipes end up adding lots of sugar, salt, and oil to replace the flavor that would be in animal-based proteins. Many people are unyielding in their conclusion: Tofu isn't worth it!

But the Japanese use of tofu has always been complementary. Instead of flat-out replacing meat, tofu is used to enhance meat dishes – in Japanese burgers or hambāgu, it's common for some of the minced meat to be replaced with tofu, to make the burger softer, absorb spices better, and make a traditionally heavy food a bit lighter and more refreshing. In soups or stir fries, instead of fully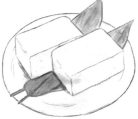

replacing the pork or chicken with tofu, Japanese recipes will call for lessening the amount of meat and in lieu adding some tofu.

In this way, consuming more tofu doesn't necessarily mean eliminating meat. Instead, it can just be about making dishes better: something a bit more nutrient-dense, healthier for our bodies, tastier to the palate, and as an added bonus, more helpful to the environment. So, if you like to eat meat, instead of being worried about eliminating the foods you love, try focusing on variety and discovering ways to add ingredients that are good for you to complement the foods you already enjoy. Sometimes eating meat is a large part of our culture and upbringing, or we simply enjoy it, and we don't need to dismiss these identities completely to find balance in our diet.

If you're not a big fan of tofu, there is a different approach to incorporating meat into a healthful and sustainable diet in Japan. Not that Japanese people don't eat meat often – in fact, I'd say that most people eat it every day – but I discovered that meat is incorporated into meals in a way that I don't often see in the United States: thinly sliced, served with vegetables.

A lot of classic Japanese meat dishes are served with thinly sliced meat – shōga ginger pork, *niku-jaga* (Japanese meat and potato stew), *nabemono* (Japanese hot pot), and *hayashi* rice (Japanese beef stew), to name just a few. If you visit the meat section in a supermarket in Japan, you'll quickly realize that the selection of beef and pork steaks is sparse. In comparison, the selection of thinly sliced meats is much greater. If you look for meat options on the menu of a traditional Japanese restaurant, even where the meat is the main, it is often served thinly sliced with an assortment of vegetables. It became clear to me that Japanese people eat meat often, but they're not eating a lot of it.

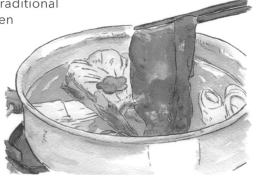

Instead of eliminating meat, the Japanese way of eating healthfully is much more focused on balance and creating dishes that use meat and vegetables together (ideally, from ethical sources).

Rather than regularly eating big steaks and chunks of meat, or completely eliminating meat from our meals altogether, it's about incorporating the flavors and fats of animal-based products to signal satiety and create well-rounded dishes that we want to eat again and again. Animal fats help trigger satisfaction cues that low-fat meals and vegetable oils can't always accomplish, an important signal necessary for those who wish to adhere to an intuition-first diet – a key principle which I, and many other Japanese people, rely on to maintain a healthy and sustainable diet.

Elimination is not the optimal diet for all of us, and we can still pursue better health and minimize personal environmental impact by making small choices in our day-to-day life. So if you're thinking of incorporating a bit more variety in your diet, consider the Japanese way of eating meat: thinly sliced, served with vegetables.

We don't need to be too worried about having to adopt a diet composed of "superfoods" or eliminating any particular food type from our diet to live healthfully. Instead try paying closer attention to the variety of fresh fruits and vegetables you eat in a day – seven a day, if you can – and ways in which you may be able to vary the other food groups present in your meals. If we can be mindful of variety with most of our meals, eating healthfully can feel less like a sacrifice and more like an opportunity to make it sustainable to our wellbeing.

This is a key to effortless lifestyle health.

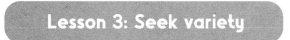

Lesson 3: Seek variety

JAPANESE WAFŪ HAMBĀGU

4 servings

Wafū hambāgu is a Japanese take on the traditional burger. Much lighter in taste and flavor, it is a great balance of sweet, salty, and a bit tangy. The tofu is a great addition because it's soft and absorbs the flavor of the sauce well, and keeps the dish light and refreshing. While it's not a replacement for an American burger, it's brilliant and delicious in its own right.

Ingredients
- 150g/5½oz minced meat (chicken, pork or beef)
- 300g/10½oz firm tofu
- 1 onion, minced
- 5g dried hijiki (optional)
- 2 tbsp all-purpose flour
- 3 tbsp ponzu
- 1 tbsp each sugar, sake, soy sauce and mirin
- 1 pack shiso leaves
- 400g/14oz grated daikon (about ¼ of a daikon)
- salt and pepper to taste
- Cooking oil (I usually use walnut oil)

Instructions

1. Press the tofu, rehydrate the hijiki, mince the onion, and grate the daikon.
2. Once ready, mix the minced meat, tofu, onion, hijiki, flour, salt, and pepper together in a large bowl.
3. Mold into patties, lightly grease the pan with oil, and cook on medium heat until they brown, flip, and then put a lid on it to let them steam for another 4–5 minutes.
4. Remove the patties from the pan and put aside. Add ponzu, sugar, sake, soy sauce, and mirin to the pan, gently stir everything together, and simmer on low. Once it reduces a bit, turn off the heat and put the burgers back in the pan to lightly cover in the sauce.
5. Plate the burgers, top with shiso and grated daikon. Enjoy!

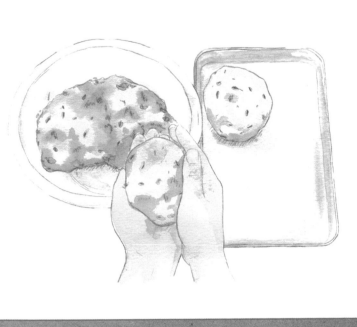

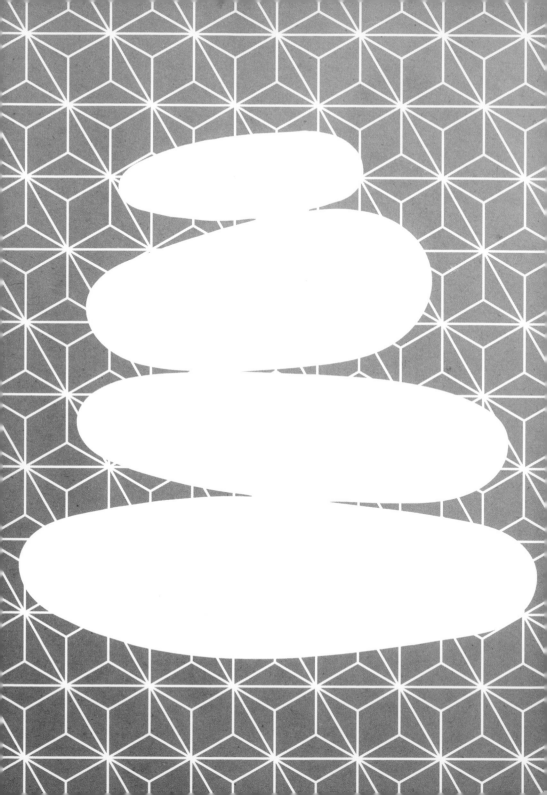

LESSON 4:
EMBRACE CONVENIENCE

There is a common misconception that healthy eating is about never taking shortcuts – that people who manage to eat well are the same individuals who have hours every day to go grocery shopping, cook in the kitchen, and make everything they eat from scratch. If you google a stock image of a person cooking healthy food, you will most likely be greeted with a photo of a put-together person chopping carrots with a kitchen knife, not a photo of a person in their pajamas, standing next to a microwave waiting for the timer to go off.

Oftentimes, however, healthy cooking can look like the latter. My mom showed me that.

One of the best resources you can look to if you want to learn how to cook quick and healthy meals is Japanese bento box culture, because if you have to make lunch for three small children at 7am every day, you need to get creative on how to cook food without the luxury of time or energy.

If you wanted to add boiled broccoli to a lunch, for example, it may seem like such a simple endeavor on the surface – it's just boiling some water and adding broccoli, right? But if you pull back the curtain you can understand why it can seem like such a hassle for someone who is under a lot of pressure for time:

1. Set a pot of water on the stove, until boiling.
2. Wash the broccoli head, cut it into florets.
3. Boil for 2-3 minutes, under tender.
4. Take a colander and drain broccoli, then serve.

This entire process is not only time-consuming, but it would require you to be attentive to your stove, and it goes through multiple kitchenware: a knife, cutting board, a pot, and a colander. Just for boiled broccoli!

Yet a Japanese cookbook for bento box lunches would never instruct you to cook your vegetables in this way. Instead, the instructions would most likely look something like this:

1. Buy a bag of pre-cut broccoli florets and put the florets in a glass bowl.
2. Add a tablespoon of water, put on a steamer lid.
3. Microwave for 2 minutes on low.

The brilliance of this process is that you wouldn't even need to be watching the broccoli to check when it's done – after you hit start, you could begin working on whatever else needs to be made that morning. The focus is less on the most graceful way to cook, and more on convenience. Because broccoli made in the microwave is still broccoli.

The first recorded instance of the bento was around the 5th century, a very basic meal called *hoshii*, meaning dried boiled rice. It was a modest bundle carried by hunters and could be steamed, re-boiled, or eaten as is.

But by the 1500s Japanese society changed, and work began to take place further away from the home, and so the first modern bento box was born. It was still considered quite utilitarian at the time – an easy way to eat on the go – but as Japan grew wealthier, people began to use it for entertaining, tea services, and when more children began to go to school, children would use it for lunch. As a consequence, eventually a core value of the homemade bento box became its nourishment: a balance of carbohydrates (which was most often rice), healthy proteins, and plenty of colorful vegetables.

Bento boxes became compartmentalized containers, a tool to visualize the balance of a meal. They would often contain a main section to hold rice, and smaller sections to hold vegetable side dishes and a protein. It made it easier for people to think about balance and how they might want to incorporate variety in a lunch.

This focus on nourishment didn't mean people didn't embrace convenience to create healthier meals – when I was young, I would sometimes watch my mom nuke an egg in the microwave in the morning because she forgot to boil them the previous night for my lunch but wanted to add some more protein, or she would take defrosted spinach and haphazardly flavor it with soy sauce and dashi in an attempt to add more greens to the meal.

Using frozen vegetables is an especially helpful approach for those who don't always have the time to plan their grocery shopping. For example, defrosting a bag of frozen edamame and flavoring it with yuzu-pepper salt can be an easy and accessible way to add an extra serving of greens and protein to a lunch with minimal effort. Use peas, brussels sprouts, carrots, or daikon on other days, and you can always have a healthy vegetable side to go with your meals.

Buying frozen vegetables is particularly helpful to those with limited time or energy for meal prepping efforts, as you don't need to worry about the food going bad and can use it when you need it. It's great to eliminate food waste and can be a solid step toward eating more sustainably.

Aside from a microwave, there is another appliance that is heavily relied on in almost every Japanese household: the rice cooker.

Why is that so? To be completely transparent, you don't need a rice cooker to make rice – rice can be made with just a pot and some water. But unlike a pot, a rice cooker distills the process down to three easy steps: rinse, add water, and press a button. There is no timer or standing over the pot to check when it's done, you can simply walk away and do something else if you want to.

Like making steamed broccoli in the microwave, the rice cooker allows the individual to save stovetop space, and perhaps more importantly, headspace. It's a form of cooking that requires no attention, which is why almost every Japanese household will have one.

What I have found out about most people's cooking habits and psychology around healthy eating is that rarely is it about not wanting to eat healthily, but rather that eating healthily can feel difficult when we're already juggling 100 other tasks in our mind. In the morning, we're rushing to get to work or school, and we don't have time to think about making a pot of steamed rice. After work, we're exhausted and the prospect of trying to make something healthy at home becomes very unattractive, even if we are the most avid of chefs. I am not oblivious to the demands of modern life, and I empathize with working parents or busy students: sometimes it would be much easier to just order some takeout or buy a ready meal on the way home.

Healthy also doesn't mean bland in taste – you can rely on certain pantry ingredients to boost the flavor of your foods, without having to resort to complicated sauces or cooking techniques to make something delicious.

But if we already have the rice cooking in the pressure cooker, and we know two other vegetable dishes we can whip up using the microwave, we can think to ourselves – okay, I just need to pan-fry some salmon, and then I'll have a full dinner. Convenience doesn't mean unhealthy; it just means convenient.

If you ever purchase a Japanese cookbook, you will notice with a lot of Japanese recipes that the ingredient list tends to only be a few lines long and the directions can be pared down to just a few statements. For example, sashimi that is only flavored with soy sauce, or miso soup that is only made with miso paste, dashi, and some cubed tofu. Yet these dishes are hardly one-dimensional in flavor.

It has become increasingly apparent to me that Japanese cuisine is often about skillfully using four key ingredients for savoriness: soy sauce, sake, miso and dashi. Almost every recipe uses at least one of them, if not several of them in combination. Why? Because these four ingredients are very rich in the flavor profile *umami*.

Savoriness, the best way to describe *umami*, is one of the five basic tastes in food. In science, this savory flavor is referred to as the taste of glutamate. The term *umami* (旨味) is composed of the two characters 旨, which means delicious, and 味, which means taste. It was first proposed in 1908 by Japanese chemist Kikunae Ikeda, but its existence was not widely accepted by the scientific community until 1985.

Umami has been applied in cooking for centuries[14] and is what *makes* the pantry staples soy sauce, dashi, sake, and miso so beloved in Japanese cooking. Just a dash of soy sauce or a spoonful of miso paste – something rich in *umami* – can make all the difference in the savoriness of our foods.

"Japanese cuisine is often about skillfully using four key ingredients for savoriness: soy sauce, sake, miso, and dashi."

And it's not just the flavor of these ingredients that makes them staples in Japanese cooking, it's also the simple convenience of them. Preserved properly, any four of these ingredients can last years in the fridge or in the pantry, and they take up little room in what cabinet space a small kitchen can spare. There is no need to spend hours boiling *kombu* kelp sheets and dried bonito to create your own dashi; it's readily available at most grocery stores or otherwise accessible online, so Japanese home cooks refer to recipes that use it again and again.

SESAME SPINACH OHITASHI

2 servings

People think that because I love preparing beautiful and delicious food that I'm above using a microwave to cook – nope! Perfect for days when you forgot to plan dinner and you think you have nothing in the fridge, this simple vegetable side dish is one you'll be glad you have saved in your recipe repertoire.

Ingredients

- 1 spinach bundle, approximately 170g/6oz fresh, or 120g/4¼oz frozen (Note: You can use frozen spinach instead of fresh! In this case, microwave until defrosted.)
- 80ml/⅓ cup of water
- ½ tbsp soy sauce
- ½ tbsp mirin
- 1 tsp dashi powder
- sesame seeds to taste

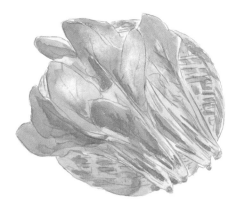

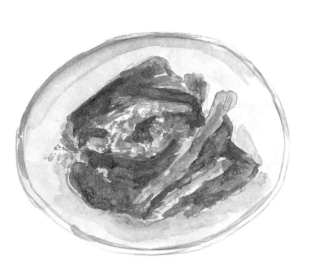

Instructions

1. Microwave spinach for 2–3 minutes, or until wilted through. Run under cold water, drain, and then cut into 5cm (2in) lengths.
2. Mix the spinach, water, and pantry ingredients in a bowl, then serve onto small plates.

SHIITAKE AND TOFU MISO SOUP

2 servings

Miso soup is a wonderful recipe to have memorized
for your repertoire because it requires so few
ingredients, and you often don't need to make an
extra trip to the grocery store to make it. I suggest
you always have some dashi powder and miso
paste at home – they're often-used Japanese pantry
staples! – and feel free to experiment with different
vegetables or ingredients to toss in.

Ingredients
- 4 shiitake mushrooms, sliced
- ¼ block of silken tofu, cubed
- 350ml/1½ cups water
- 1½ tbsp red miso paste
- 1 tsp dashi powder

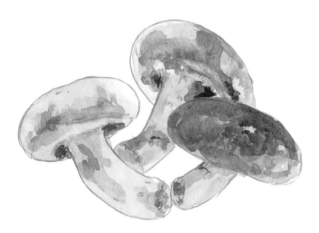

Instructions

1. On medium-high heat, combine shiitake mushrooms, tofu, water, and dashi until simmering, but not boiling.
2. Once the shiitake mushrooms are cooked through, reduce to low heat and add the miso paste, stirring to dissolve. Serve into small bowls and enjoy!

Note: If you don't cook with shiitake mushrooms often, a good option is to use dehydrated mushrooms instead!

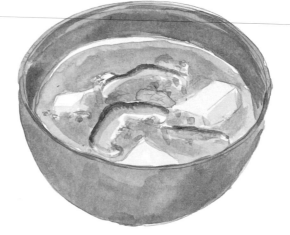

Rarely do we ever dislike healthy foods themselves, but often our perception is that healthy eating habits are at odds with a busy lifestyle, which is why many individuals have difficulty adopting them. We aren't left with lots of energy to cook after a long day at work, and takeout meals of salad and grain bowls can get boring day after day, not to mention taxing on the wallet.

But cooking for yourself matters because it's about being in control of what goes in your body. Preparing your own foods puts you in touch with what you eat and how it affects your body in ways that pre-prepared or takeout meals can't.

Cooking not only nudges us to pause and think, "What does my body want or need today?" and make meal decisions accordingly, but it also allows us to reflect on a meal more thoughtfully afterwards. If we feel it was a bit heavy for our stomach, we may think to ourselves, "Next time I'll add less olive oil", or if we observe that it left us feeling a bit jittery, we may make a note to use less sugar in the sauce and add more fibrous vegetables. We begin to connect the dots on what went into our bodies and how it affected it and learning from this cycle we can more closely find a balance of eating that allows us to enjoy what we eat, but in a way that still serves our health.

"Cooking for yourself matters because it's about being in control of what goes in your body."

When we rely on pre-prepared foods too often, we lose this visibility into our meals and hence find it difficult to understand our unique needs for food, and therefore can't adjust our way of eating accordingly. We don't get to choose how sweet or salty something is, and we can't choose to make a dish with less oil or more fiber. It's a compromise we can make on occasion to enjoy a wonderful meal at a restaurant or celebrate with takeout at the end of a particularly stressful day, but when we do it too often, we just don't know what our body needs because we aren't exactly sure what's in a particular dish. Yet when we adopt home cooking, we naturally learn to adopt intuitive eating as well.

This insight on the value of cooking has shown me the value of investing in anything – from prepared miso pastes to an expensive rice cooker – that makes the process of home cooking more relaxing and enjoyable, rather than time-consuming and stressful. Because that's the key to maintaining a healthy diet: enjoying the process and foods you put into your body. If you can accomplish this with fruits, vegetables, and nourishing proteins and grains, then your health goals – whether that be weight loss, immunity, or longevity – will naturally fall into place.

So instead of 10,000 hacks or "clean-eating" shortcuts, we should be thinking about investing in our health for the long term, and the tools to help us get there. A sustainable, healthy lifestyle necessitates loving what you eat and the process of making it, and this means investing in the tools and ingredients that make home cooking easier, less expensive, and taste that much better in the end.

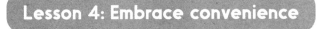

Lesson 4: Embrace convenience

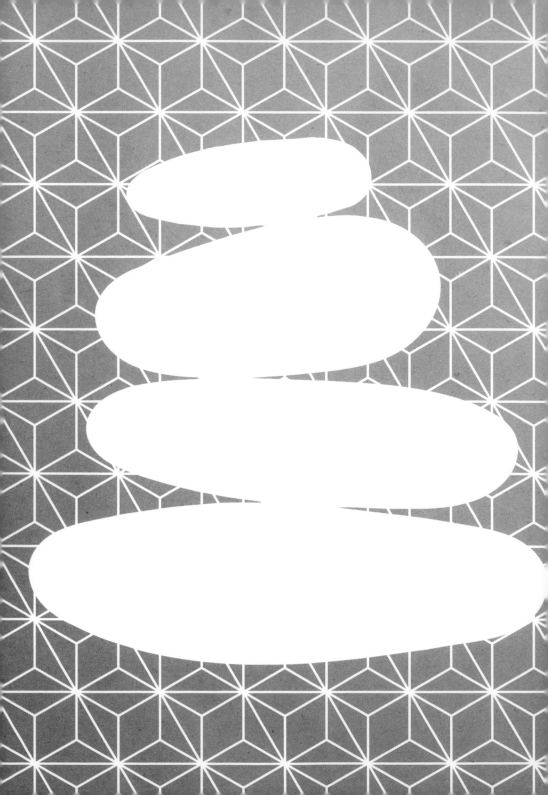

LESSON 5:

PURSUE QUALITY

Japan is a very food-centric culture, so much so that when you pose the question "What do you want to be when you grow up?" to an elementary school classroom, chances are that quite a few of them would answer that they want to be a restaurateur or chef – in fact, pastry chef regularly makes it into the top three career choices for elementary school students, and is often in the top 10 among high school girls.[15]

Bakeries and pastry shops in Japan are notorious for being consistent in delivering high quality, beautiful desserts. Even if you walk through any major train station there are at least several vendors offering amazing desserts to buy on the spot. Food is such a big part of the culture in Japan that it's customary to bring back sweets or artisanal local snacks to your friends or family when you go on a trip, or if you are about to go into a meeting with a business partner you will often offer them some sort of *wagashi* or Japanese confectionery gift to share amiability.

Food is also a big part of entertainment. The American television show *Iron Chef* was originally inspired by a Japanese cooking show of the same name and concept, a timed cooking battle between guest chefs revolving around a specific theme or ingredient. As well as competitions, many popular Japanese television shows are of celebrities walking around a city and visiting famous cafés and restaurants, trying out food and giving their review of a particular menu item, or visiting a farm or fishing area and learning to cook with a regional delicacy item. People love to talk about food, learn about it, and discover new places to go with friends and family.

But the fact that there is a big food culture in Japan does not mean that most of these people lead very unhealthy lives; perhaps ironically, I would argue that Japan's love for indulgent food is what keeps it so healthy.

The final lesson surrounding healthy eating may best be understood through how we perceive one term: indulgent. A small perspective shift, but it can be the difference between "healthy living" and "always on a diet".

I remember my grandmother coming home with a fancy box wrapped in a shiny pink ribbon one day. She excitedly announced to us that afternoon that she had a nice surprise waiting for us after dinner, a really special and decadent treat to look forward to, so we should probably not eat too many snacks during the day.

The box was huge and felt heavy - a chocolate cake perhaps? I secretly hoped it would be chocolate cake. It was too heavy to be a Japanese dessert, and she immediately put it away in the refrigerator, so I assumed it wasn't going to be cookies or a pound cake of any sort. I was very excited to find out what was inside, so I diligently spent the day eating modestly so I could enjoy whatever treat she had prepared for us to the fullest extent.

When time for dessert rolled around, I could hardly wait. My grandmother made us take out the nice dessert plates and the teacups normally reserved for guests, so I knew it was something special. She made my siblings and I gather around the table, and made the big reveal …

I was confused: they were mangoes.

I think my grandmother took my speechlessness as that of delightful surprise and began to explain how a friend from Okinawa had sent her these mangoes as a gift. With each mango costing about $40 (£33), her friend had sent a box of four to share with us. It was the strangest gift I had ever heard of at the time – artisanal and expensive mangoes – but then it hit me: the sweet, tropical, and fruity smell.

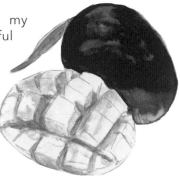

Almost like a perfume, the aroma was so strong I was shocked that it was coming from the fruit. I carefully lifted one out of the box and felt how heavy and ripe it was. Perfectly bright red, smooth, and not a single blemish on the skin: it was the most beautiful mango I had ever seen in my life. I watched with fascination as my grandmother expertly cut open the fruit, mesmerized by the amount of juice and the ease with which she sliced through the flesh. When I finally got the chance to pierce it with my own fork, it was almost like pudding, and the sweetness melted in my mouth before I had the chance to bite into it. I had already forgotten about wanting chocolate cake.

What do you think of when someone mentions "indulgent food"? If you thought of something along the lines of overflowing milkshakes, candy, burgers, and fries, you think like the majority of Americans, or perhaps western countries in general. It can be confirmed with a very quick google search, as you will most likely be greeted with images of gooey cheeses, dense chocolate cakes, thick burgers, and piles of golden fries.

But while indulgent food is often associated with unhealthy food in the US, this is not necessarily the case in Japan. The top online rankings of Japanese luxury foods[16] aren't super sweet or calorie dense, and there is a relatively weak correlation between "unhealthiness" with how indulgent something is. When you mention indulgent food to a Japanese person, the foods they think of will probably be along the lines of fresh seafood, artisanal fruits, fancy meats, seasonal vegetables, and delicate *wagashi* Japanese confectionery.

Indulgence doesn't necessarily mean it has to be expensive either; other factors that are highly prized are the particular seasonality of a certain fruit or vegetable, the locality from where it is harvested, or even the history of its creation. Cheese from Hokkaido – a region famous for its dairy products – is considered indulgent because Hokkaido is well-known for its lush farming conditions with its cool climate and plenty of wide and green pastures, making it an ideal environment for cows to produce high-quality milk. *Hōjicha* tea from Kyoto – a region famous for its green tea – is considered indulgent because the region has a long history (over 800 years!) of producing, inventing, and perfecting the growth and drying of green tea leaves. One time, I was gifted a box of fresh squid! It was a famous delicacy from the Saga Prefecture in Japan, a town called Yobuko, which is well-known for

being able to catch lots of fresh squid. Even if it is not very expensive or Instagram-worthy in size, the idea of local, historical, or seasonal can be considered indulgent. What these foods always have in common is a strong focus on quality.

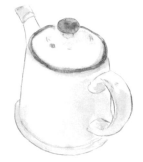

This difference is key because it shapes our understanding of what joyful food is. When unhealthy, large, and abundantly sugary or calorie-rich foods become our version of what "treating ourselves" is like, trying to eat healthy seems like a choice of deprivation. It means we're always on a diet, always holding back on joy. This idea of depriving ourselves not only makes a diet unsustainable, but it can even lead to shame and stress, or habits of "diet-breaking" and binge-eating.

There is also a notable difference in portion size when it comes to indulgence. In the American version, plates are often overflowing, ice-cream sandwiches can barely contain themselves, and burgers and fries are piled up high. In this sense, quantity can be equated with being better, or more indulgent.

But in the Japanese version of indulgence, sizes are often relatively moderate. It would be a stretch to call it a small amount, but it's clear that quantity is not as much of a defining factor. Instead, there is a much stronger focus on presentation, plating, and delicate garnish: a smooth, bright red mango wrapped in high-quality paper, or a piece of tuna sashimi sliced at the perfect angle to show off its shiny color.

This focus on quality rather than size does not just encourage moderation; it also encourages us to become more mindful around our meals. There is a good reason why there are few Michelin-star restaurants where the average mealtime is 30 minutes or less, because when meals are delicately balanced and carefully plated, we are psychologically primed to pay attention and thus take our time eating.

When we focus on quality – of food, but also experience – there is no forced counting of the number of times we chew or trying to stay mindful of the flavors we taste. We just naturally slow down as we redefine the feeling of treating ourselves. It's no longer associated with feelings of being overstuffed, but with taste and experience. Eating in moderation becomes not only easy, but natural.

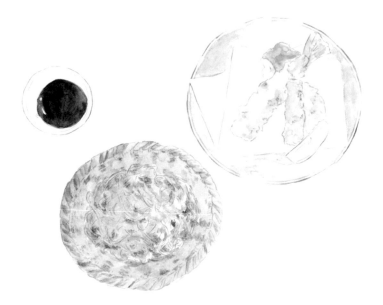

When we understand that food that is high quality, seasonal and delicious to us is what really makes something indulgent, then healthy eating can become one and the same with the idea of treating ourselves. Eating seasonal, sweet mangoes can become our idea of indulgent eating, not ice cream. Smoked and grilled fresh seafood becomes just as appetizing as a big burger.

This does not mean that sweets or fried foods are never considered indulgent in Japanese culture – Japanese people are not inherently different, and they enjoy these foods as much as any other human being – but Japan has a slightly different relationship with these traditionally "unhealthy" foods, which allows the culture to be very food-centric while still maintaining general health among its population.

There is a popular narrative in the dieting world that has made many people equate living healthfully with a lifestyle that is highly restrictive. It associates meals of skinless chicken breast and steamed broccoli with discipline and control, whereas luxurious meals of creamy pastas or sweet desserts are associated with guilt, over-indulgence, and sometimes even laziness. But how could enjoying good food make anyone lazy? Telling someone to eat stricter meals and to cut out desserts is usually well-meaning advice, but it's not very useful.

"Eating healthfully and eating indulgently should not be seen as two mutually exclusive lifestyles."

Most diets fail not because the science behind diets is wrong, but because dieting is not a long-term solution – there is always a point we want to stop. But if we focus on a way of eating that doesn't rely on deprivation, individuals find much more long-term success because they are able to keep up with it forever: what we enjoy, we don't change.

Eating healthfully and eating indulgently should not be seen as two mutually exclusive lifestyles. We can design lives where we enjoy the foods we love and never worry about the calories, while still living the healthiest life we could possibly imagine. Because yes, the two ideas can and should coexist. For once you can combine an indulgent diet with a healthy one, meaning that a healthy life feels less like a chore and more like a wonderful pleasure of life.

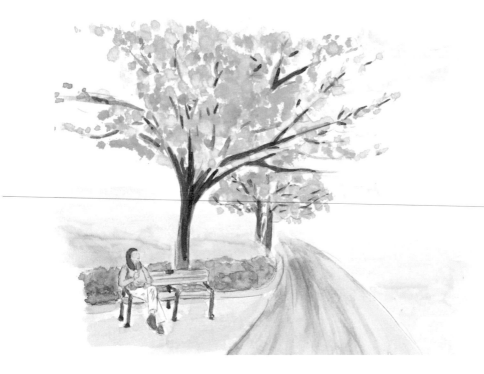

Lesson 5: Pursue quality

PILLAR 2:

MOVE

What is the purpose of exercise? When you speak about exercise with most people, it usually comes up in two different contexts: if you're younger, you may be thinking about it as a way to improve your physical appearance, and if you're older, you may be thinking about it as a form of disease prevention.

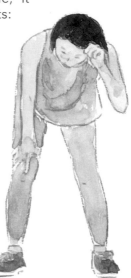

Neither lens is inherently wrong, but it feels like an uninspiring way to think about something that can be an amazing asset to our lives.

If you were to open a health app or check the screen of a treadmill, you might think that the most important thing about exercise is the number of calories you had burned or your average heart rate during the session. We may not think we pay much attention to these details, but compounded regularly, eventually when we visualize the meaning and importance of exercise it feels less holistic to our entire wellbeing, and more boxed to a certain number.

Calories burned to lose weight to look better in our jeans. High average heart rate to prevent heart disease. It may seem like the natural way to think about the purpose of exercise, but upon closer inspection it's a perspective rooted in fear and punishment – that if we don't regularly engage in some sort of exercise, we'll suffer negative consequences. It's no wonder that so many people have a complicated relationship with it.

We shouldn't feel at fault for thinking of exercise as a chore rather than a gift, for even with the best of intentions, this is how many of us have learned about the importance of exercise. We don't talk about how it's important because it improves our confidence, boosts our mental wellbeing, or is simply another way to feel joy. Instead, when speaking about exercise most individuals in western education systems are simply told that we should be getting at least 150 minutes of moderate aerobic activity or 75 minutes of vigorous aerobic activity a week,[17] and that if we do so we will lower our risk for most diseases. A guideline provided by the CDC, we have learned to speak of exercise like a medical prescription rather than an opportunity for joy.

I didn't think much of it at the time, but reflecting on it, it's such an odd way to encourage exercise. When we learn about exercise through the point of view of a doctor's prescription, many of us begin to associate it with the act of going to the gym, getting sweaty, or the feeling of muscle soreness the day after. That if we are not deliberately "working out" that somehow it doesn't count, and exercise becomes colored by terms like "no pain, no gain". We begin to believe that exercise that doesn't push us in some way is almost like exercise that isn't worth doing.

But talking about exercise in this way can make us more weary than excited about moving our bodies.

I remember one time I was speaking with someone that I was health coaching for, and she described how she didn't have enough time to work out the past few days because she had spent the weekend shopping in the city. She was feeling a bit stressed out that she was perhaps backsliding on any health progress that she had made and vowed that next weekend she would make sure to carve out time for a workout.

Before I properly replied, I first asked her to pull out her phone and show me the number of steps she had taken over the weekend. It was over 15,000 steps on both days!

"Being able to expand our scope of what exercise can look like is important."

Do those steps not count as exercise? Of course they do! It may seem obvious to us in retrospect, but it is not uncommon to be tunnel-visioned into a belief that exercise worth doing necessitates sweating, soreness, going to a gym, or wearing workout clothes. We associate strenuous physical exertion with meaningful exercise, but there is benefit to be gained from movement outside this scope as well. Something like going shopping with your friends on the weekend is a completely valid way to enjoy moving your body.

Being able to expand our scope of what exercise can look and feel like is important because exercise that we don't enjoy doing is exercise that we fail to continue. Instead of being stressed or preoccupied with the minutiae of what counts or doesn't count, we can find movement which is tailored to our values, joys, and needs, rather than a textbook prescription. Through this perspective is where we find a way to exercise that we are willing and wanting to do for the rest of our lives, a way of moving that allows us to live our most fulfilling and meaningful life.

In this part I may challenge your idea of what exercise looks or feels like. I will discuss the elements of it that we should be paying attention to, so it is something sustainable, natural, and enjoyable in our lives. This is why I call it movement; to hopefully nudge one to see that movement is something as old as time, and that we don't need to regard it as a separate workout that must take place outside of our daily life if we choose not to. Because at the end of the day, exercise that is worth doing is simply any kind of movement that may benefit our wellbeing - physically or psychologically - everything else is just noise.

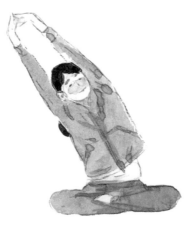

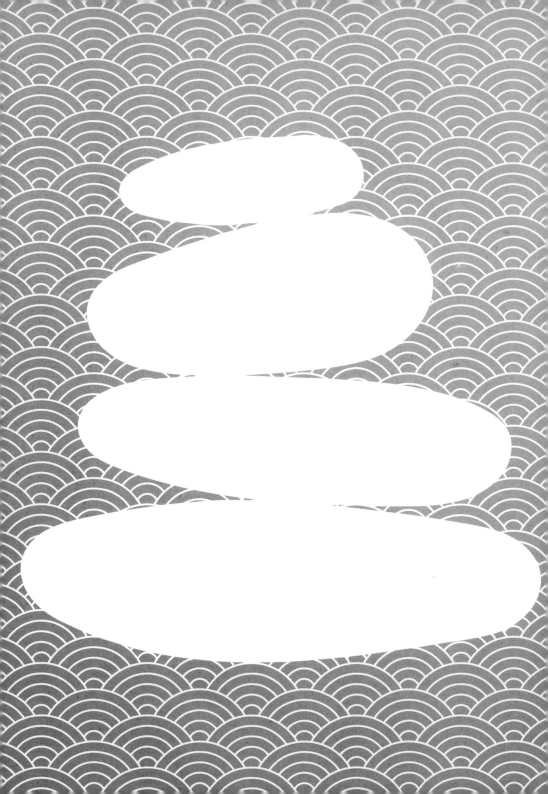

LESSON 6:

EMBED WHAT FITS

In the US, I'm often bombarded with images and ads of fitness culture. Athleisure is the craze, and it seems that most people are members of gyms like Anytime Fitness, Equinox, or Gold's Gym. Any decent hotel or typical college campus has free access to a gym, sometimes even offering workout clothes for rental. It's the land of Alo Yoga and the birthplace of CrossFit. The most successful online influencers write about fitness, and it's not uncommon to see someone share their workout on social media as they would their food.

But in contrast to that, for a country that is a leader in longevity and has very low rates of obesity, you might be surprised to find that there is not much of a workout culture in Japan. Athleisure is not a big thing, and not many people have a membership to a gym. People rarely use their lunch break for a gym session, and those who do are probably seen as exercise zealots. In a 2018 Rakuten Insight survey of 1000 Japanese citizens aged 20-70, about half of those questioned revealed that they barely exercised;[18] about once a month or not at all. Citing not enough time or simply that they don't like exercising that much, most people just didn't see working out as part of their lifestyle. What's going on here?

If you take a closer look at what exercise means to the modern person, most people will equate exercise with working out. But movement is not just going to the gym or wearing fitness wear, and is not necessarily about lifting weights or going on 10km (4 mile) runs either. The exercise we need might not have to be the kind we carve out time for as a separate activity; perhaps it could be the kind of exercise that is already weaved into our lifestyle, such as walking.

What the above results show is not that exercise isn't important to be healthy, but that in Japan's approach to moving, most individuals aren't going to the gym to lift weights or going on long runs to find it. Instead, what most Japanese people are doing is simply walking. Japanese adults walk an average of 6,500 steps a day,[19] with males in their 20s to 50s walking nearly 8,000 steps a day on average, and women in their 20s to 50s about 7,000 steps. Nagano, a rural prefecture in Japan, was able to reverse their high stroke rate by incorporating over 100 walking routes[20] into their city. In the early 1980s the prefecture had one of the highest rates of strokes in Japan, but after establishing these walking routes and encouraging locals to use them, by 2014 they were ranked number 1 in life expectancy in Japan, with the average woman living to 87.2 years and the average man to 80.9 years.

Most Japanese citizens live in very walkable cities where public transportation is convenient, safe, and affordable, and not many households own cars. Greater Tokyo has one of the world's most extensive urban rail networks, reportedly serving about 40 million rides daily[21] – consequently, when most people go to work, they walk. When people go grocery shopping, they walk. When people go out for dinner, they walk. It's an activity adopted every day by every generation; like breathing, walking is a part of daily life.

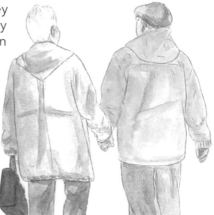

I love working out, and don't doubt the advantages of a good sweat to boost our physical and mental health, but fitness culture can feel overwhelming for those who aren't used to it, and too much can perpetuate cycles of shame and guilt. It can make us believe that reaching and maintaining a healthy weight is only available to the dedicated ones who consistently lift weights and are making enough time for daily runs. The truth is, though, impactful exercise doesn't require intense exertion, sweating or hours logged outside of our usual routine.

> "Impactful exercise doesn't require intense exertion, sweating, or hours logged outside of our usual routine."

Consider the things that you do anyway. In my earlier example, someone who enjoys shopping can go to the mall or into the city to window shop instead of spending that time browsing online. If you enjoy eating out, instead of driving up to a restaurant for lunch you may choose to go to the park or go on a short hike and host a picnic outside. If you enjoy thrills and games, plan for an outing to go to an amusement park with some friends. You probably won't even notice it until the end of the day, but you will often find yourself having walked a considerable distance.

You can also make micro-adjustments in your daily routine like choosing to go to the grocery store on days you have more time, rather than having your groceries delivered, or if you work in a city or someplace with accessible sidewalks, you may choose to commute to work by train or bicycle instead of a car on days where the weather is nicer. It doesn't need to be every day and it doesn't need to be every time, but by being mindful of ways we can incorporate movement in activities we would be doing anyway, we can make exercise feel less like a chore and more like a natural part of our daily lives.

CLASSIC TUNA-MAYO PICNIC ONIGIRI

2 servings

Onigiri is a classic staple to bring onto hikes and picnics. Easy to carry and easy to share, it's one of my favorite foods to make because it's adaptable to so many different flavors and great to make use of any leftovers. In this version I share my favorite flavor, but feel free to use whatever filling is available to you!

Ingredients

- 300g/10½oz room-temperature cooked rice
- 1 sheet dried nori (approximately 18cm × 20cm, or 7in × 8in)
- 70g/2½oz can of salted tuna
- mayonnaise to taste

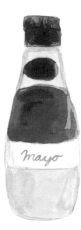

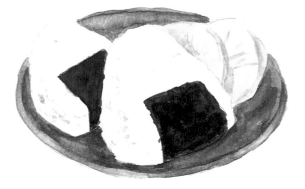

Instructions

1. In a glass bowl, mix together the canned tuna and mayonnaise. Make sure to remove excess water from the tuna!
2. On a sheet of saran wrap, add ¼ of the rice and spread thinly. In the middle, place ¼ of the tuna-mayo mixture.
3. Gently mold the rice in the saran wrap, so it takes on a rounded triangular shape. (Note: If you would like to skip the saran wrap, you can use wet hands to mold the onigiri!)
4. Wrap in a sheet of nori and enjoy!

The kind of movement that is valuable to our bodies can sometimes be quite subtle. I remember talking to my grandfather when I brought up how he had pretty good mobility for someone quite old, in his mid 80s. He climbs the stairs to a fourth-floor apartment, goes on daily walks several kilometers at a time, and is always sitting up straight during meals. He doesn't have any back, knee or hip problems, and his posture might just be better than mine. When I commented on his mobility he smiled and nodded proudly, "It's because of *Makko Ho.*"

Makko Ho is a stretching system developed by a Japanese man named Wataru Nagai,[22] who once suffered a stroke and found his body paralyzed. His doctors said he most likely wouldn't regain his mobility, but he decided to work on his rehabilitation through stretches based on Buddhist poses (his father was a monk) and called it *Makko Ho*, which means "the practice of facing things". It worked.

Based on his own experience he ended up writing a book, and the exercise quickly found popularity among the Japanese elderly and those interested in anti-aging calisthenics. It's a very basic form of stretching – only four different stretches! – and is believed to help keep your body healthy and youthful.

Makko Ho is a type of stretching that is used to help create stronger and more balanced synergy between the bones and muscle groups, and improve physiological improvements in the human body. It does this using the theory of the meridian system, which was popularized in Japan by Tokujiro Namikoshi, who first studied Chinese qi bodywork and Japanese medicinal and martial art practices to treat his mother's rheumatoid arthritis. He claimed that the body was connected through a network he described as "meridians", and by placing pressure on specific areas near the joints this helped to stimulate the body's adrenal glands (organs involved in the production and release of hormones), which would naturally release cortisol and help the body heal itself. His shiatsu therapy later gained worldwide traction, and the foundation behind the therapy – the meridian system – later inspired many other practices.

The wonderful thing about *Makko Ho* is that even if you're not a physical therapist, and don't quite understand the exact science or mechanics behind how the practice is beneficial to your body, one thing will become very clear to you as you engage it: small steps, when practiced consistently, make great differences.

As I found myself dedicating three minutes of my morning and evening to stretching, I found that the good habits impacted other areas of my life. I felt more refreshed and inclined to go for a walk outside during the day. I felt myself growing more flexible, and motivated by my progress I would challenge myself to hold deeper positions for longer periods. When I had the time, I would often stretch for more than 3 minutes, simply because it felt so good. Setting aside that time relaxed me, and it also built my confidence.

"Small steps, when practiced consistently, make great differences."

I used to think for exercise to be beneficial, it meant I had to break a sweat and feel worn out afterwards. But I have since realized that even if movement is simple and asks for only three minutes of your time, consistency goes much farther than you'd think. It reminded me that moving your body is not really about gaining more muscle or endurance - it's about regaining your quality of life.

For me, *Makko Ho* embodies the idea that we don't need to make stretching and moving into an elaborate hour-long endeavor. We don't need to be pushing ourselves to make a stretching session worthwhile; what we really need is to keep it consistent - and if short and simple helps, that'll be more than enough to keep your body mobile, strong, and youthful for years to come.

HOW TO PRACTICE *MAKKO HO*

Practice these stretches for 3 minutes each session, twice a day: once in the morning, once in the evening. Please note though that it's hard to do these straight out of bed or if you've been sitting for a long period of time! Warming up with a few squats and sit-ups first makes the stretching a lot more comfortable.

1. Hold each of the following three stretches for 40 seconds.

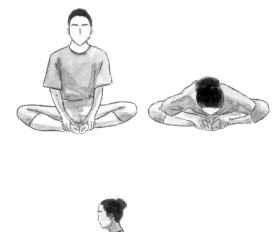

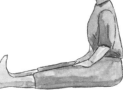

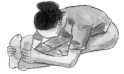

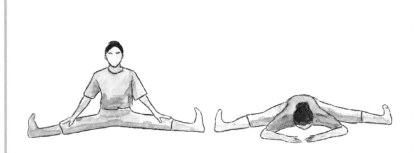

2. Hold the next, and final, stretch for about a minute. This is the most difficult stretch, and so if this does not feel comfortable for you, please don't push it! Continue to do light squats and the first three stretches until you become more comfortable.

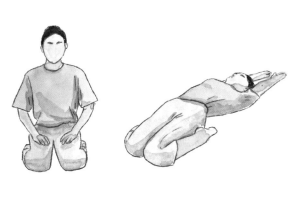

In Japan, the value of daily stretching – even for just a few minutes a day – is nationally recognized as a way to not only move our bodies, but bring people together. If you ever get the chance to visit Tokyo, I suggest you visit one of the city's best-kept, and perhaps slightly quirky, secrets. Every morning, if you go to Ueno Park at 6:30am, you'll find hundreds of people gathered at a plaza – appropriately named Rajio Taiso Square – to do something very simple: stretch.

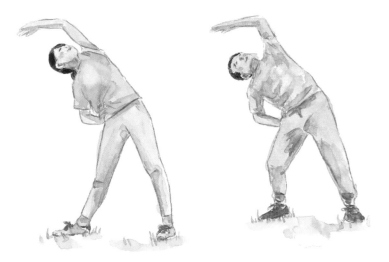

Rajio taiso, or radio calisthenics in English, is a popular stretching routine developed back when the radio was the most popular form of media. Every morning the *rajio taiso* program would play on the national news network: a 3-minute simple exercise routine designed to get the muscles moving, blood flowing, and start your day refreshed.

Created with both the children and the elderly in mind, the movements were meant for everyone, at any level. Eventually radio calisthenics became routine in schools, workplaces, and government offices. If you grew up in Japan, you would be familiar with *rajio taiso* like an American would be familiar with their national anthem, except instead of a song it is also a stretch.

Radio calisthenics is regarded as a rather outdated activity today, but the legacy of the national practice continues. The stretch is still performed at school sporting events and local volunteer communities, and the Ueno Park *rajio taiso* community brings in about 300 individuals every morning, a mix of newcomers and veterans, with the longest attendee said to have been going for over 40 years.

What are the health benefits to such a short, simple exercise? There must be something of value if hundreds of people are committed to it every day, and for so many years over their lives.

In general, stretching is valuable to our health and wellbeing because it keeps our muscles flexible, which is necessary to maintain a full range of motion in our joints.[23] If we don't regularly stretch, our muscles become tighter and shorter, which can pose risk for injury and pain when we try to engage these muscles and they are unable to extend fully.

Take, for example, a rubber band: if we spent a few minutes every day gently pulling it and stretching it out, it would extend much further, and we would be able to extend it with ease. But if we were to neglect stretching this rubber band, eventually it would become very stiff, and if we were to try to pull it, it would not stretch as far, and may even snap if we were to do it too suddenly. Our muscles work in a similar way, where we need to consistently stretch and extend them out to make sure we can use our limbs and body without restraint, and reduce the risk of injury.

In the modern world, many of us spend much of our day sitting, but this position can actually lead to tightened hamstrings, which makes it harder for us to extend our knees properly and makes running or walking more difficult. Prolonged sitting also results in tightness of our hip flexors and puts a lot of pressure on our back muscles.[24] If we were to suddenly extend these tight muscles by carrying something heavy or climbing up a steep incline, we may injure our back or leg muscles, and find our body in pain for days afterwards. These kinds of injuries are particularly a concern for older individuals, where a fall down the stairs or trip on concrete could be fatal. While we don't need to fear sitting, what we do need to do is make sure we regularly stretch to undo this tightness and keep our body mobile and free. Remember, you could have the best sitting posture possible, but there is no position that humans are meant to hold for more than several hours – it is much more important to occasionally move around and stretch.

There are many different kinds of calisthenic stretches we can do, but there is a reason why *rajio taiso* was so influential to Japanese culture. The value of it is quite subtle, because I won't argue that the calisthenic exercise burns many calories, is great for quick muscle building, or will train you to do the splits. But its greatest asset is that it is so unassuming, it's primed for becoming a habit.

"Making it a habit, instead of a chore, is the easiest way to stay fit and healthy."

Like brushing our teeth or combing our hair, we don't think about habits because they're so ingrained into our routine. It's only a few minutes, but if we didn't do these things every morning the consequences on our wellbeing would be significant. It is the same with movement, and the reason why consistency is more important than any one exercise regime or workout protocol. Making it a habit, rather than a chore, is the easiest way to stay fit and healthy. It doesn't need to be an hour-long endeavor, but if you can find a few minutes every day to move and stretch out your body, those small habits can go a long way.

In the US, there is a popular notion of "go big or go home", and that anything that is worth doing should be executed to the fullest extent. While I recognize the value of putting your entire spirit into everything you do, it's a mindset that can make the prospect of challenge and change difficult – and every step counts, so we shouldn't dismiss the value of going slow and small. Exercise is not an all-or-nothing game, it's for the rest of our lives – so why not take our time with it?

Like how eating healthfully doesn't need to be eating only salads, healthful exercise doesn't need to be only working out at the gym and breaking a sweat – maybe what is right for you is something much simpler. Not all of us can spare hours at the gym for exercise, nor do all of us want to. All exercise needs to be is a form of movement that we are willing to embed in our routine and daily life.

Lesson 6: Embed what fits

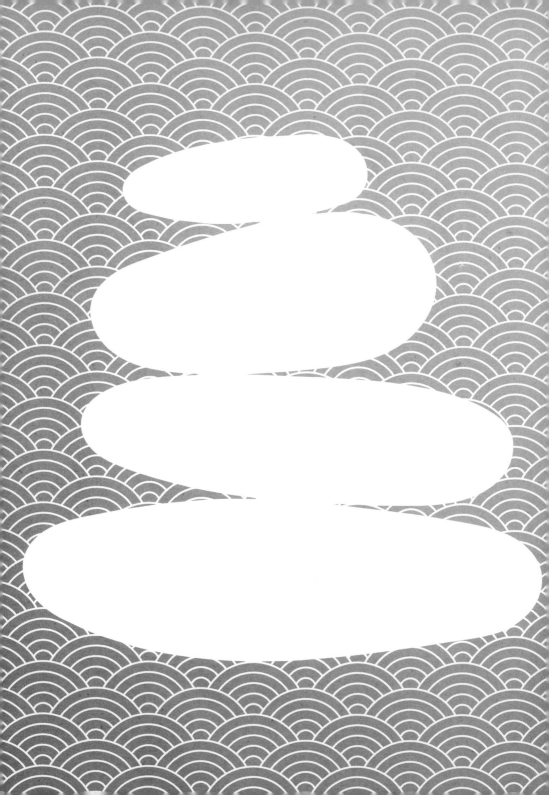

LESSON 7:
FOLLOW JOY

In the modern world, much of the purpose of exercise lies behind goal-setting. Milestones like reaching a certain weight or wanting to be able to complete "Couch to 5k" are common, and because we hold a goal-oriented mindset toward exercise, we grow to be attentive toward a formula rather than our own intuition. People often want to know what they should be doing for exercise to meet a certain goal – what is the most effective workout for weight loss? How do I build flat abs? What should I be doing every day to be able to run 5k? A half-marathon? We seek 30-day workout challenges and daily training plans that promise to get us to our goal by the end, putting priority on the outcome rather than the journey.

I believe in goal-setting and think it is an effective and important way to motivate ourselves and hold ourselves accountable. The concern is that while I believe there is value in guidelines and a routine in instilling important health habits, sometimes we become so focused on the goal that we lose sight of the bigger picture. It is not uncommon for someone to become so concerned about the goal that finding a form of exercise that they enjoy and brings fulfillment to their life becomes of secondary importance. But how can we expect to continue to do something we dislike for the rest of our lives?

The number of times I've heard someone tell me they want to be able to run a 5km (3 mile) race, but then tell me a few minutes later that they hate running, still surprises me. But this is how we have learned to think about exercise, that the goal is more important than the journey, and that we should will ourselves into certain workouts even if we aren't particularly inclined toward them. Like taking on a career that we hate to become wealthy, we forget that there are enough options in the world where we can find a job that we enjoy, fits our values, and can help us make enough money to live our dream life. Exercise is important but the world is creative enough that we can find a form of movement that we enjoy, fits our values, and can keep our body healthy and strong enough that we want to do it for the rest of our lives.

Exercise that we do not enjoy is exercise we do not continue. But if we are mindful of what we need at a certain moment, and approach it with a positive attitude, the prospect of maintaining the habit of exercise becomes much easier – almost natural.

I understand why many people have difficulty viewing exercise through the lens of joy, when they feel that they must be "good" at it or somehow already "fit enough" to engage in exercise that they are curious about. When I lived in the US, I remember the first time I had to describe to my parents the school sports team try-out process, and how I didn't want to go because I knew I wasn't as good as the other kids and wouldn't make the team anyways. They looked at me incredulously, because at such a young age – I was only 13 years old – I was already counting myself out of an activity. To them, it seemed impossible that a child would be counted out of a sports team because of their skill level.

"Exercise that we do not enjoy is exercise we do not continue."

The idea of try-outs and team cut-offs felt normal to me at the time, but upon closer inspection it sows confusion when you are told the importance of exercise but then are barred from it because of skill or experience. Couldn't you just join a sports team because it would be good for your wellbeing? From a young age we are told that we have to be good at something to engage with it, but if you haven't played before, how are you to get better at it? Growing up in this environment, many of us are shaped to understand the endeavor of adopting a new exercise habit as fearful and intimidating, rather than curious and exciting. It tells us we value skill when it comes to movement, and that it is not always something we can just enjoy for the sake of enjoyment.

My parents grew up in a Japanese school system, where even high school sports don't have team cut-offs. Everyone is allowed to participate and is given the opportunity to learn and get better, no matter what experience level they play at. This doesn't mean it's an "everyone gets a trophy" kind of world – only the most skilled and dedicated players get to play in real matches or find themselves on the pitch, but everyone is allowed to come to practice. You get to participate in the drills, scrimmage with others, and put yourself in a community where you might not be the most-skilled player, but you get to have fun.

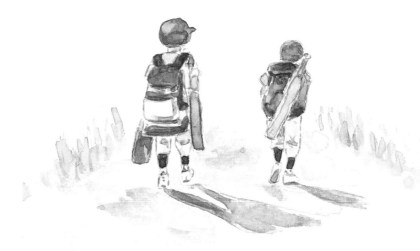

BENTO BOX TAMAGOYAKI (JAPANESE ROLLED OMELET)

2 servings

An *undoukai* bento wouldn't be complete without a small side dish of *tamagoyaki* nested inside the box. Delicate and soft, and just the subtlest amount of sweet, it's delicious hot, cold, or room temperature. After a day running around outside, nothing tastes better!

Ingredients
- 3 eggs
- 1 tsp sugar
- 1 tsp dashi powder
- 1 tsp neutral oil

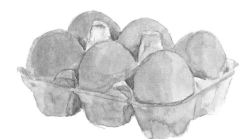

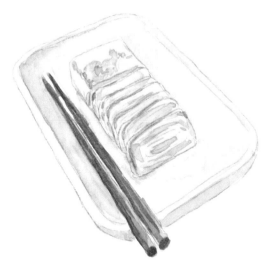

Instructions

1. Thoroughly mix the eggs in a bowl without foaming them up.
2. Slowly add the sugar and dashi powder.
3. Heat the pan to medium-high and add oil, using a paper towel to coat the entire surface.
4. Lower the heat and pour in ⅓ of the egg mixture, covering the entire surface.
5. Once the bottom layer is cooked, slightly fold in the right and left side toward the center to create a rectangle.
6. Then fold the far end of the rectangle in 2in, and continue to roll it toward you. It should look like a rolled-up crepe.
7. Push the roll back to the far end of the pan and pour in another ⅓ of the egg mixture, lifting the roll to get the egg mixture under as well.
8. Fold the edges in toward the center and roll the rectangle in again.
9. Repeat the process with the remaining egg.

It's easy to say that exercise is for everyone, but the Japanese school system makes it evident: no matter who you are, you are built to move and you can learn to get better at it.

One of my favorite days of the Japanese school year was Sports Day or *undoukai* (運動会), a day where the entire school is split into two teams, red vs. white, and everyone competes against each other in a variety of games. Some are a bit more serious, like track and field, but others are there for simple fun, like potato-sack racing. Parents may come to watch their children compete and cheer them on, and whether you are an athlete or not, the purpose is for all the students to have fun and become closer as a school.

Growing up overweight as a child, attending my first *undoukai* was something that had intimidated me. I was not fast or strong, and I was fairly certain that my classmates would not welcome my participation for I didn't have much to offer in terms of athletic ability. I couldn't help my team win, so why should I even try? But when the competition is tossing bean bags into baskets, jumping through hula hoops, and rolling around comically large rubber balls, it did not matter if I was fit or not. My teachers and classmates would cheer me on the entire time, and it was all done in the mindset of fun – I was running and jumping, climbing and chasing, and by the end of the day I would be so sun-baked exhausted that I would find myself about to fall asleep on the train ride home. After every Sports Day, I would think, even unathletic me can have a great time!

"Moving our bodies is all about good fun."

Undoukai is an important part of the Japanese education system, and anyone raised within this system will be familiar with the tradition. It's so significant that *undoukai* doesn't end with our student years – Sports Day is a recognized national holiday and once a year, adults get the day off from work to celebrate sport for what it is: a fun way to move our bodies and be part of a community. Exercise is not seen as something we should "just be doing", but as something that we should be celebrating. Moving our bodies is all about good fun.

There is a short proverb in Japanese, *jiyu-honpou* (自由奔放), that highlights the importance of being able to live in a way that is not bound by the rules and customs of the world, but one that is informed by your own needs and desires. It recognizes the value in doing things in accordance with your wishes, and not what is prescribed by society. To live *jiyu-honpou* is to live by your own intuition – and what is one of the most powerful forms of intuition we have in our toolkit? Joy.

We often associate joy with pleasure, leisure, and entertainment – that it is largely optional, and that it doesn't belong in the realm of things that we should or need to be doing. Yet joy is a powerful form of intuition, and it can tell us something about what is good for us – moving our bodies doesn't need to feel like a chore; it can be something that we enjoy and look forward to. Intuiting with joy can nudge us to make choices that are best for our wellbeing.

There is no one best way to move our bodies, and even if there was, it would be safe to assume that the exercise we do as a teenager is not the same kind of exercise we would expect to do when we are in our 80s. Instead, the best kind of exercise changes as we grow older, even month by month, or day by day. A study published in 2000 found that when participants were asked to exercise for eight weeks, variety in workouts significantly helped individuals adhere to regular exercise.[25] These findings were also supported by a separate study published in 2020 which found that highly active adults also tend to regularly vary their exercise.[26] It helped decrease boredom and maintain enjoyment, making adherence feel less like a chore and more like something they wanted to continue.

You may not need to read about formal research to believe in the benefit of variety in exercise. If you were to look at interviews with global centenarians and what they do for exercise, you will probably not find one clear answer. Okinawan centenarians are famous for their active lifestyle, but they credit a plethora of things that they do regularly to their good health. Some regularly engage with tai-chi or yoga, others credit their garden hobbies, and some may simply attribute it to how they sit on the floors in their home, and how this helps them improve their strength and mobility. There is rarely one exercise regimen that overshadows them all, for what is best for us is simply what we enjoy.

Sometimes the appropriate thing to do for our wellbeing is to go for an intense workout, to sweat out the stress, and feel exhausted by our efforts. It can be refreshing and reinvigorating to the spirit to wholeheartedly immerse yourself in a physical activity. But other times the appropriate thing to do for our wellbeing is not the intense workout, but instead something slower and more relaxing for the body's muscles, like a slow walk or a stretching routine. Rather than a silver bullet solution, our exercise needs are constantly changing, and the key to sustainable and beneficial exercise is being able to follow your sense of intuition - joy - for what is best for you in any given situation.

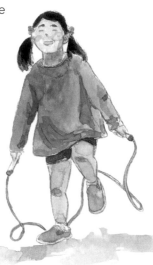

I can empathize with how it can be quite difficult to trust our intuition in terms of what our body needs, especially if we are new to exercising, and don't know if we are doing the right things or if we are doing enough of it. In turn, we like to come up with numerical values, protocols, and routines to guide us. I believe these are great and powerful tools that shouldn't be dismissed, but when we lose sight of our humanness and treat ourselves like programmable computers, exercise slowly morphs into the arduous and uninspiring task that will eventually burn us out and force us to quit. However, when exercise is done in the right spirit, instead of exhausting us it will make us feel stronger, more confident, and more energetic.

So be mindful of your joy. Some days you might want to sweat and feel exhausted, other days maybe not. Some days you might want to exercise in peace and quiet, other days you may prefer to be with company. It doesn't need to be routine; what movement should ultimately be is what you feel like doing in any given moment. We don't need to be particularly skilled at exercise or perform it for the sake of being able to reach a certain physical milestone. In essence, exercise is just about moving our bodies, and we should see it as something joyful and fun before anything else.

> "Exercise is just about moving our bodies, and we should see it as something joyful and fun."

It can be a tool for social connection and camaraderie building, or it can be a space for mindfulness and releasing the thoughts that circle your head during the day. It can be the time when you get to focus on music and let out your stress, or it can be a time when you get to be outside and connect with nature. It can be fun, it can be spiritual, it can be calming, or it can be energizing. There is no need to be driven by fear or guilt, for there are many joyful purposes to exercise we can focus on. Once we find that purpose we resonate with, exercise will never have to exist as a chore to us again.

Lesson 7: Follow joy

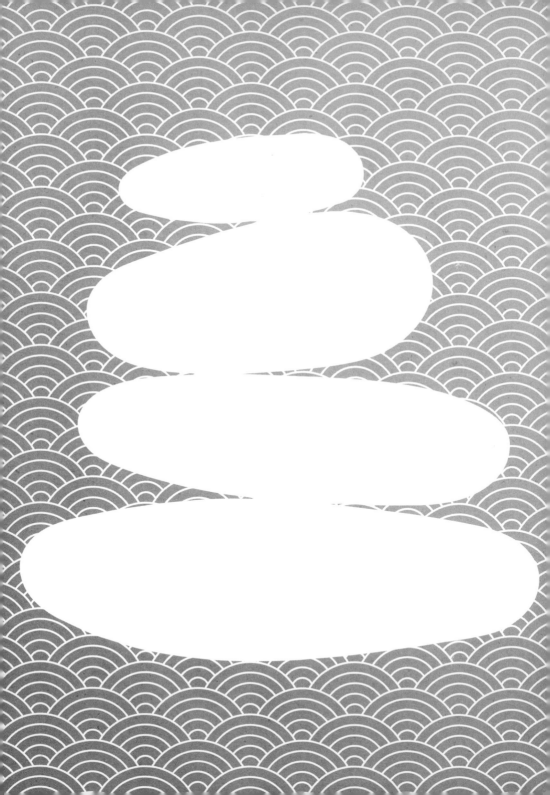

LESSON 8:
MIND YOUR ENVIRONMENT

Imagine being stuck in a room for two weeks, and having to work, eat, entertain, exercise, and sleep in the same 100sq ft or 9sq m bedroom. If that is not enough to make someone go crazy, it is enough to make them incredibly bored.

That was me during the spring of 2020.

I had not caught coronavirus myself, but I had taken an emergency flight from New York to Tokyo to be with my family when it became clear that this was not a simple several-week stint and was going to be a lasting pandemic. On entering Japan I was required to self-quarantine at home for 14 days, unable to leave the apartment or even go outside for fresh air. For two weeks my life was contained within the walls of my apartment, mostly spending time in my small bedroom.

I was quarantined, but I was healthy, so I wanted to make sure that I had a way to move my body. In terms of exercise, I thought it wouldn't be a very difficult two weeks because I had my yoga mat with me and was quite comfortable doing YouTube workouts for exercise. Even if I could not go on a run or visit a gym, being able to stretch and strength train at home felt like it would be enough. But let me tell you – while I would quarantine again if I had to for the safety of the people around me, despite my best efforts it was a very uninspiring experience.

While it has been proven in multiple studies that exercise can help relieve stress,[27] I found that exercise couldn't deliver me much relief when my bed, desk, and walls were inches away from where my yoga mat was laid. My room in Tokyo was much smaller than my room in the United States, and while I technically had enough space to do the exercises, it just wasn't an effective environment for me to enjoy moving my body.

Home workouts have their own benefits in convenience and comfort and can be just as effective as going to the gym, but just because we can physically do it at home does not necessarily mean that is the ideal environment for us to move our bodies. What is in our vicinity matters when it comes to working out – we should be in a space that is conducive to a mindset focused on exercising and moving our bodies, not be distracted or stressed by our environment. Finding joy in movement is not just in the activity, but in the environment in which we do it as well.

Luckily one of the most scientifically backed effective spaces to improve our mood and motivation is one of the most accessible – the outdoors.

If you've ever gone on a mountain hike or a leisurely stroll in a woody park, you have probably experienced one of the best ways to improve your sense of wellbeing and peace. Perhaps you found the presence of towering trees to be soothing, or the sounds of birds chirping to be uplifting. You may not have had a word for what you were experiencing at the time, but this phenomenon is well-known and highly supported in Japan: shinrin-yoku or forest bathing.

During prolonged periods of stress or chaos, there is this human draw to not just the quiet, but often specifically to nature. We want to see the sky, feel grass, hear rivers, and feel fresh air because these elements bring us peace. Just being there almost feels like we are healing ourselves. *Shinrin-yoku* is this practice of spending time in nature and is clinically recognized as an effective form of healthcare in Japan. In fact, the term *shinrin-yoku* was conceived in 1982 by the Japanese Ministry of Agriculture, Forestry, and Fisheries,[28] and can be formally prescribed by doctors, similar to how one might be prescribed medication.

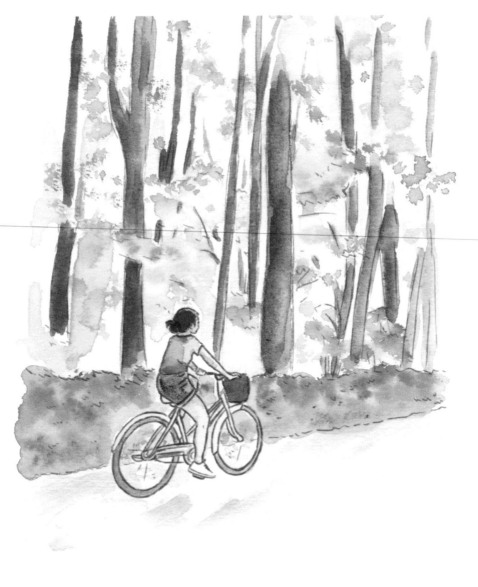

Dr Qing Li, a professor at Nippon Medical School in Tokyo, is often referred to as the world's foremost expert in forest medicine. According to his research, only two hours of being within nature can lead to a host of benefits like reducing blood pressure, lowering blood sugar levels, improving memory, and boosting the immune system.[29] His studies have even shown drops in the stress hormone cortisone, and an increase in average sleep by 15 per cent of the participants.

"Finding joy in movement is not just about the activity, but in the environment in which we do it."

Dr Li asserts that the most effective way to practice forest bathing includes leaning into our five senses and paying attention to things in our environment that we may usually feel distracted away from. He believes that we should be mindful of the details we tend to take for granted – such as touching the bark of a tree, smelling freshly cut grass, or really listening to the rustling of leaves in the breeze – to heal ourselves from the inside out. Even examining the different shades of green when sunlight peeks through the canopy or taking a moment to smell the fragrance of soil, is enough to bring measurable changes to our health. Seemingly simple details, but this methodology has been shown in studies to boost one's immune system,[30] lower levels of mortality and illness,[31] increase self-confidence,[32] and help patients cope with high levels of stress, anxiety, or grief.

A separate study conducted in 2019 found that those who spent at least two hours a week in nature experienced a boost in both their physical and mental health.[33] Interestingly, it was not significant whether that time was in one big chunk on the weekend or taken in short intervals.

It may be of little surprise then that people in "Blue Zones", places in the world where people experience particularly low rates of chronic disease and high rates of longevity, tend to have very

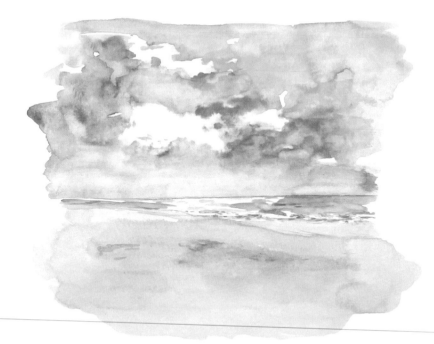

nature-rich lifestyles. Okinawans from the village of Ōgimi, one such Blue Zone, are famous for their nature-rich lifestyle full of gardening and time in the sun, factors which have been shown to help keep their hearts healthy, bones strong, and maintain a positive attitude toward life.[34] In fact, amusingly the people there live so long that by the entrance to the rural village there is a small stone marker that reads: "At 80, you are merely a youth. At 90, if your ancestors invite you into heaven, ask them to wait until you are 100 – then, you might consider it." [35]

Like eating well and getting exercise, spending time in nature is just as healing to our quality of life no matter our culture, generation, or the era we live in. We think more clearly, find peace, and boost our spirit in the outdoors – that's an incredible power. Because as much as we've grown to spend more time indoors and live a lifestyle communicated through digital means, humans will always marvel at the joys of fresh air, the beauty of watching plants grow, and the strength of moving water when we get to feel it in person. We come back to it because it heals us, and while we may not all have backyard access to a forest or ocean, even a walk in the park or an open window can work wonders. There is no medicine quite like it.

"Humans will always marvel at the joys of fresh air, the beauty of watching plants, grow, and the strength of moving water."

This is not to say that exercise that is done indoors is always of lesser quality or benefit, as I believe that going to the gym, doing home workouts, or finding other ways to be active indoors is still incredibly beneficial to our health. Instead, it is simply to say that when looking after your health, remember to get exercise, but don't forget to be mindful of your environment. Finding exercise that we enjoy is not just about what activity we choose to do, but where and when we do it can be just as impactful.

Lesson 8: Mind your environment

JAPANESE SHISO PESTO

Makes 1 small jar (about 8oz/240ml)

Fresh herbs serve as a great way to add not just
a few extra vitamins and minerals into our meals,
but also as a reason for us to get outside and start
a garden. A particularly popular herb in Japan is
shiso – also known as perilla leaf in English
– a popular culinary herb grown in many
home and school gardens. It's fast to
grow, resilient, and easy to maintain as
a plant, and its bright and sharp smell
adds a wonderful flavor addition to
many dishes. Shiso pesto is one
of my favorite ways to use it!

Ingredients
- 80g/2¾oz shiso leaves
  (100 leaves)
- 60g/2¼oz pine nuts
- 1 clove garlic
- 120ml/4fl oz/½ cup extra
  virgin olive oil
- 1 tsp salt
- parmesan cheese to taste
  (optional)

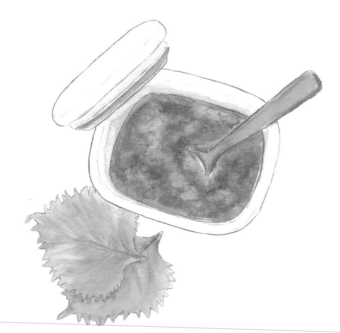

Instructions
1. Rinse the shiso, then drain.
2. Toast the pine nuts in a dry pan, just enough so they begin to smell nice.
3. In a food processor or blender, add all ingredients and blend until smooth.
4. Serve with pasta, bread, cheese, or tomatoes – enjoy!

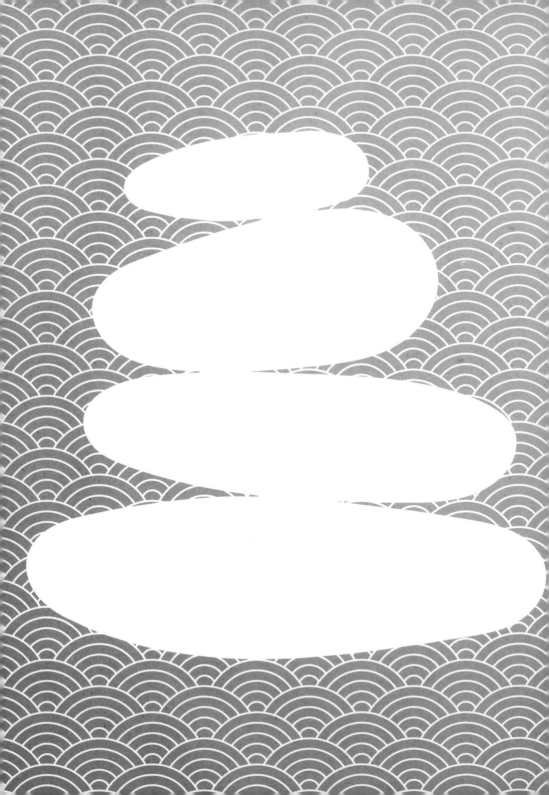

LESSON 9:
EMPOWER YOURSELF

Choosing what works for our lifestyle, what we enjoy, and where we engage with movement all have a large impact on our adherence to exercise, but perhaps one of the most significant determinants of our ability to adopt a lifestyle exercise lies in our motivations.

I'd like to revisit our motivations, for it is fairly common for people to start exercising because there is something about their life that they are unhappy with. Perhaps it is a perceived shortcoming of one's appearance or a critical note by their doctor that they are not doing enough to protect their health. It is commendable and admirable for one to take it into their own hands to improve their life, but the beginning of this journey is not always easy. Many people begin exercise with a rather dispirited mindset that feels disparaging of one's self worth, rather than one of confidence.

I personally was motivated by weight loss when I first embarked on my health journey, but coming out of it I realized that my weight actually played a lesser role in how I felt about myself than I had expected. I will grant that it was an effective motivator for weight loss, hence why so many health and fitness ads tend to focus on this component, and it is true that losing weight may improve one's physical and mental health. But reliance on appearance as a reason to exercise can be rather counter-productive for our wellbeing – it can make us stressed, self-conscious, and preoccupied with working out, rather than being mindful of why moving our bodies is good for us in the first place. The internal dialogue can be a lot harder to shape than the actual physique.

Many of us understand how preoccupation with the body can negatively affect our wellbeing, and may have tried to find body acceptance amid concerns about our own appearance. However, this is difficult because obsession with the body can feel inescapable, like it's everywhere in the world. We get ads for it, are subtly nudged by television and movies, and are bombarded with content that puts physique at the forefront of its messaging. Despite our best efforts to block and report ads or follow content that is less uninviting, it can be exhausting. But one day I found a little relief in a piece of clothing that allowed me to not pay too much attention to the body: the kimono.

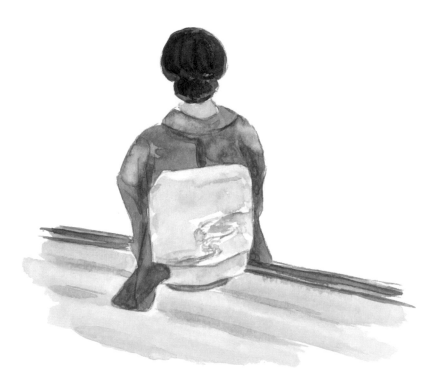

In traditional kimono dresses for women, the goal is to wear it in a way where the body looks like a tree trunk: no curves, just a straight, thick pole. Why? Because wearing a kimono is not about the body's appearance, it's about showing off the kimono's fabric and pattern, and you want it to look strong, crisp, and clean. Instead of worrying about how to make your legs look longer, your waist look narrower, or your arms look thinner, when you wear a kimono you ask yourself questions like: How can I match the fabric's color to the season? What color obi band matches the dress? What hair accessories would complement the color accents in the pattern?

From a western perspective – a perspective historically informed by corsets for women and heels for men – clothing has often been seen as a way to enhance the body, to show it off to others. But Japanese kimono tradition had shown me a perspective where the shape of the body was of very little importance when it came to the art of dressing yourself. Instead, you could simply focus on how you felt in it.

"Focus on the journey rather than the outcome."

I think body positivity is a well-intentioned movement, and I wish more people would love and feel beautiful in their own skin, but the pressure to feel great in your body can push you to take care of your body in ways that make you unhappy - working out to exhaustion, forgoing your favorite foods, hiding yourself in photos - and paradoxically, sometimes the effort to love your body can make you resent it. But if we can adopt a perspective where we simply don't pay attention to the way the body looks, we can find contentment with what we have, and focus on the journey rather than the outcome.

So instead of carrying shame or being motivated to exercise out of guilt, try shifting this narrative slightly. We are not broken and there is nothing wrong with us. All we wish to do is empower ourselves with a lifestyle that makes us feel strong and confident, and lets us lead a meaningful and fulfilling life. As long as we pay attention to the person inside, that is all that we need to accomplish this.

I would like to recognize that while it is important for us to take care of the body, it is not always something that feels exciting. As much as I champion putting joy at the forefront of this, it is expected for there to be moments where it feels tiring, boring, and perhaps even a bit tedious. Yes, taking the time to look after your body can be a bit like maintenance work sometimes. But maintenance work is not something to be avoided, and it doesn't necessarily have to be viewed through reluctant eyes – in fact, with the right spirit it is the most enjoyable form of work that we can participate in.

If you've ever visited Japan, you may be impressed by the amount of heart and effort that goes into any sort of job. Phenomenal customer service is not limited to high-end luxury shops and hotels – if you walk into any regular store, you will likely be greeted by an employee who will politely welcome you in, bow to you, and rush to help you as soon as they realize you need assistance. Their uniforms are clean and their appearance clearly cared for. The shelves are put together, the products aligned and organized. Floors are mopped, windows are wiped down, and when you exit the store, the employees will say thank you, smile, and bow to you until you are a considerable distance from the exit.

The idea of putting your best foot forward – *ganbaru* – is one that is highly valued, no matter what context you employ it in. Whether you're CEO of a large corporation, a professional athlete, or simply a participating member in a school group project, we find that those who exemplify principles of *ganbaru* are not just highly respected, but they enjoy the work much more than those who decide not to feel optimistic about what needs to be done.

Ganbaru is not necessarily a physical effort. It doesn't mean putting in many hours of work, overtaxing our bodies, or pushing ourselves to a psychological limit, which eventually leads to burnout. Exhaustion is not admirable and should not be sought after. Instead of an external effort, what *ganbaru* really refers to is the spirit of doing our best - something that most people experience as simply a positive attitude, a mindset geared toward optimism. Instead of shuffling through the drudgery, by embodying the spirit of *ganbaru* we can transform the prospect of something that may feel arduous at first into something much more engaging.

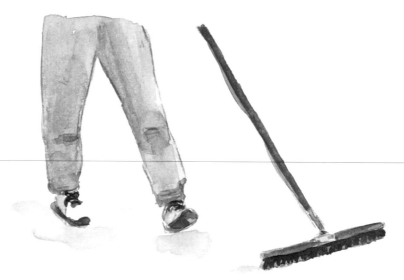

So instead of going into exercise with the mindset of having to simply log in a set number of minutes or miles, try going into it with an attitude of optimism - how can I make this interesting for myself? What can be fun? How can I uplift those around me or my community? - and perhaps we can drastically change what the prospect of exercise means for us. Moving our bodies doesn't need to constantly be about how to most efficiently reach our health goals; we can enjoy ourselves throughout our relationship with it.

"Moving our bodies is about ... finding a way to make our lives more fulfilling, meaningful, and empowering."

Rather than letting ourselves be motivated by shame or frustration, we can take on an attitude of empowerment when it comes to our exercise. Instead of focusing on what is yet to be done or accomplished, we can put focus into the journey and go into it with an open attitude – experiment, discover what you like and don't like, and see what aligns with your values and fits your lifestyle best. Moving our bodies is not about changing what we don't like about ourselves, but finding a way to make our lives more fulfilling, meaningful, and empowering. We don't need to wait until the finish line to feel this way; we can do it from the very beginning.

Lesson 9: Empower yourself

PILLAR 3:

REST

If you've grown up in a competitive environment, you have most likely been taught that rest is something that can be negotiated. Whether that be directly or indirectly, many of us have learned to see that studying for the exam is more important than getting to bed, or working late into the night is more applaudable than clocking off at dinner time. At times we may have found ourselves in a sort of odd competition of "who had the least sleep last night", or that we should commend people who are always busy with something. Many of us have grown to associate busy-ness with importance, even at the cost of rest. But what does that lack of rest then cost us in terms of wellbeing?

"Without proper rest, everything is suddenly more difficult."

It is important that we invest in this pillar of our health, for if we fail to pay attention to it, our efforts in other aspects of our wellbeing will at best be less effective, and at worst, be counterproductive. For example, consider how effective a workout is after pulling an all-nighter. The workout itself would be exhausting, and the benefit you'd receive would be marginal as you are unable to perform to an adequate level. Additionally, you would be placing unnecessary stress on your body and your muscles would be unable to recover, increasing your risk of injury. Lack of sleep can also cause you to make poorer food choices,[36] and can lead to anxiety and depression.[37] Without proper rest, everything is suddenly more difficult.

But I'd like to add that encouraging people to get proper rest is not as simple as instructing people to sleep earlier at night or installing nap pods in the office. There is a very large psychological component to be considered with rest, for it is also about rest in the mind: being able to disengage from worrying, intrusive thoughts, or emotional distress. When we are struggling with our mental health, it not only makes it more difficult to fall asleep, but it becomes more difficult to stay asleep – even if we are physically exhausted, sometimes our minds will not allow us to rest. This is insomnia, a condition that 10–30 per cent of the world population struggles with,[38] and almost a third of the UK population reported struggling with in 2017.[39]

To find psychological rest, some may engage in self-care activities like taking bubble baths or playing video games to detach from work and distract from the stresses of life. Through this lens, rest is understood as "non-working hours" or time spent doing something for leisure. Books, television, watching videos, gardening, and listening to music tend to fall into this category. However, it is possible for us to engage in leisurely and calming activities, yet still not feel rested after them. While these activities are temporarily distracting, sometimes they can lead to us feeling more stressed and anxious, feeding into a dangerous cycle. For a lot of people, this is best described as procrastination.

Being tasked to write a book, I know this feeling particularly well now.

After I signed my book contract, I felt excited and energized by the writing project. I would daydream about how it could change lives and inspire people, that I could write something that would be useful to anybody, anywhere, and for generations to come. Personal health has always been a passion of mine, and already having lots of experience writing about the topic, I couldn't imagine myself being really stumped. I've also always been a good student, and trusted that I could meet my deadlines with ease.

To prepare, I did what I typically did when planning for a long-term project: I printed out my schedule, broke down my milestones into smaller tasks, chose some dates to work, and let myself follow the plan.

All I had to do was follow the plan.

If only I would just follow the plan.

Some days I would get as close as sitting down at my desk, opening my laptop, turning off all my notifications, and having a four-hour timer set on my phone to commit to the time frame to write. But the most curious thing would happen: I would find that the room was too hot and the air conditioner needed to be turned up, but as soon as I sat down again the room would get too cold and I would have to put on some socks. Then I would find that I accidentally chose an ill-fitting pair of socks – were they always this uncomfortable? – and I needed to find my fuzzy socks to get comfortable enough to write.

Okay, you got your socks and you're comfortable now. Let's use this time to write something about Japanese breakfasts. Then I'd think that my breakfast this morning was kind of small, so I should probably snack on something. I'd suddenly remember how writing while hungry is no good for creativity – that I had definitely read that somewhere once – and that I might as well treat myself to the Starbucks across the street so I can finally get into the right headspace to write.

At this point you may be familiar with what happens: You go to Starbucks, you take a nap, you realize two hours have passed, and you conclude that today is just not the day to write and you decide that tomorrow you will put in more time to make up for it.

The irony was not lost on me that as I put more pressure behind writing about balance and wellbeing, the more I procrastinated, and I would increasingly find myself stressed and up at night as my deadlines approached. Eventually I admitted to myself: Yeah, my inability to write probably doesn't have much to do with the temperature of the room or the kind of socks I am wearing.

Much like healthy eating or getting exercise, people often blame the individual (or themselves) for procrastinating, and insist that they just need to put their head down and get it together. But procrastination is not an issue of self-discipline or laziness; underlying our inability to move is an unaddressed fear and anxiety. We feel unready to act so we distract ourselves in an attempt to give ourselves a break, but this distraction is unsuccessful in helping us

feel rested, so we dig ourselves into the distraction even further –
and the cycle continues.

With this in mind, instead of simply equating rest to physical rest or
the act of "non-work", it may be more helpful for us to define rest as
engaging in an activity that allows one to feel refreshed or recover
strength. Activities that allow us to replenish our curiosity, passion,
and enthusiasm for our interests and goals is what rest is – it's an
act of increasing our bandwidth for life.

When defined in this way, sometimes acts of rest may not appear
to be acts of rest. What I have outlined in this chapter describes
not necessarily how to get more sleep or how to work less, but
how to calm the mind and soul, and how this can in turn help us
to refresh and recover. By expanding our scope for what rest can
be, we can identify not just distractions, but acts that energize and
heal us so we can live our most fulfilling lives. Once we define this
as our foundation for rest, everything else about our health and
wellbeing will feel much more effortless.

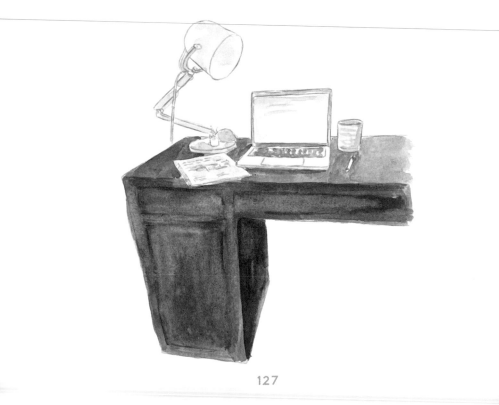

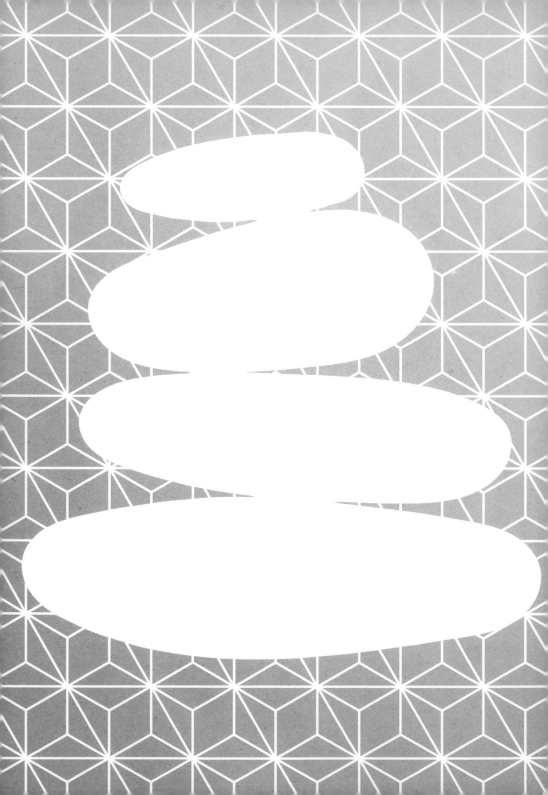

LESSON 10:

SLOW DOWN

What value is there in slowing down? In the US, it is perhaps more common to meet individuals who like to move fast, and in big and bold moves, rather than those who see taking their time as the appropriate way forward. Personally, after moving to New York it only took me a day to pick up on how nobody waited for the crosswalk lights to turn to green, and that the traffic lights here were treated more like suggestions than rules. Everybody's always in a rush to somewhere, and an extra minute saved is seen as an extra minute that can be put to work elsewhere.

This mindset stems from a society rooted in fierce competition, and to keep up many people believe that we need to be doing more and in less time, with some people going as far as abusing prescription medication to get more done. In the US or UK, it is not uncommon to hear of students taking non-prescribed ADHD medication – stimulant drugs like Adderall and Concerta which help increase focus – to try and get ahead in the classroom,[40] and more and more early-career workers are reporting reliance on these drugs to improve their productivity and output in the workplace.[41] If having the energy and time to work more is not possible within the natural bounds of human capacity, some people see nothing wrong with using drugs to extend that.

It is easy to empathize with this need to push ourselves to a psychological and physical limit to get ahead, and it doesn't take much leaning into the world to understand where it's coming from. Competition starts at an increasingly younger age, cram schools are the norm and not the exception, and spending your 20s working 12-hour days is not unheard of. People pushed to their limit will often go to the extreme for a solution – because when taken over the edge, extreme solutions seem like the only viable option.

Yet I believe the real solution to our perceived need to work more lies somewhere less revolutionary. There is a story that I enjoy that I discovered inside *The Four Agreements* by Don Miguel Ruiz. He narrates the tale of a man who wished to rise above human suffering and find enlightenment.

The man in the story wanted to find someone who could guide him to his goals, so he went to a Buddhist temple to find a master.

> *"Master, if I meditate four hours a day, how long will it take me to transcend?"*
>
> *The Master looked at him and said, "If you meditate four hours a day, perhaps you will transcend in ten years."*
>
> *Thinking he could do better, the man then said, "Oh, Master, what if I meditated eight hours a day, how long will it take me to transcend?"*
>
> *The Master looked at him and said, "If you meditate eight hours a day, perhaps you will transcend in twenty years."* [42]

The man was so focused on reaching the outcome of transcendence as soon as possible that he missed the point of how meditation helps one reach it.

While not all of us have transcendence in our list of life goals, many of us have probably faced this similar sentiment of wanting to achieve something as quickly as possible. For example, when learning a new language, if we become so transfixed on wanting to achieve fluency as soon as possible that we commit to studying vocabulary and grammar at a desk for several hours a day, we tend to struggle more as we forget the value of making friends in the new language or learning more about the culture it's used in. Similarly, learning an instrument can feel the same way – if we become so focused on improving our skill that we commit to spending hours in a room practicing alone, we forget the teaching value of performing in front of others.

This sense of urgency often stems from the belief that we can't use the language until we're fluent, or that we can't perform in front of others until we're skilled, but if we spend all of our time only focusing on the mastery we hope to achieve instead of taking our time and enjoying the smaller milestones along the way, we can lose sight of the bigger picture and become tired, desolate, and frustrated by the journey rather than energized by it. Rather, taking our time learning in smaller increments can not only make it more enjoyable, but can make achieving our goals easier.

Competitive society values people who win and excel, and we are raised to believe the good life is the hardworking and busy life. In the US, it's common to find people who constantly want to be doing more and to a grander scale compared to the people around them, and that bigger is always better. But our desire to be busy and productive all the time is unsustainable, for if we fail to also see the value in slowing down, we meet burnout, exhaustion, and sometimes find ourselves becoming indifferent toward that which we worked so hard.

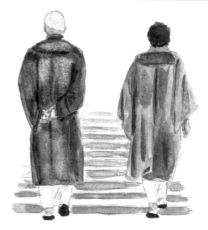

In Japan, a trend of chronic overwork and competition has led to a phenomenon known as *hikikomori*, or young people who become recluses in their parents' home and refuse to leave their room for months or years at a time. In China, many individuals have turned to *tang ping* or a "lying flat"

movement – a popular social protest by young Chinese people that describes rejecting marriage, having kids and getting a job, and instead participating in society as little as physically possible. These are not weak-willed people who couldn't make it; it is a very natural response for any person when overworked to a point of exhaustion. We end up so tired that we just want to be left alone.

This is why the skill of slowing down is so important. Ideally it can be encouraged by schools, workplaces, and a society that allows room for slowing down without the repercussions of falling behind. More likely it will start from a place where individuals take it into their own hands to identify their values and priorities, and ease the pressure on themselves independent of what others expect of them. It may be difficult to shake off the need to always move as fast as possible, for not many things in the modern world see the value in slowing down. New products, services, and even entertainment seem to be made for the sake of being faster, more efficient, and more instantly gratifying. But the world did not always value speed and efficiency – most evidently, we can still find glimpses of where slowing down is valued in a traditional art form.

Traditional Japanese arts like *sado*, the ceremonial preparation and presentation of green tea, or *shojin-ryori*, the traditional dining style of Buddhist monks in Japan, are notoriously lengthy processes. Yet this is neither a concern nor a drawback, for they are activities that are intended to be done at a leisurely pace. The mindfulness and care with which they are conducted is precisely what makes the art so valuable to the artisan and the audience. The joy is in the slowness.

A Japanese tea ceremony can be as short as 45 minutes, or a full-length formal affair can be as long as four hours. It is a practice that was introduced to Japan by Buddhist monks, and is a drawn-out process designed to help one leave the material world to experience harmony and peace in the spiritual realm. Every movement and gesture is intentional, and carefully choreographed to help the guest reach this realm – nothing is to be rushed and no step is to be unplanned. Even the angle at which objects are placed and the pace at which things are done are thought through, because these smaller details help one become more present in the moment rather than distracted by our thoughts.

"The joy is in the slowness"

Shojin-ryori was similarly brought to Japan by Zen Buddhist monks in the 13th century. It was believed that not only tea but also food was an effective way to align the body, mind, and spirit. The dishes in shojin-ryori are centered around soybeans, seasonal vegetables, and locally available plants, and are traditionally designed to be very labor-intensive dishes – many shojin-ryori dishes require repetitive grinding, boiling, chopping, and waiting. This is intentional, for it was thought that the focus and demand required of the preparation, compared to how quickly it could be consumed, could teach individuals patience and gratitude. It was the process that was important, not the dish itself.

Reading about these long and arduous traditional arts, we may find ourselves reluctant to try experiencing it for ourselves – a four-hour tea ceremony seems like it would be difficult to sit through – but when we are primed for a mindset of total immersion, it is not too difficult. What these arts enable is a state of mindfulness where you are so fully immersed in an activity that nothing else seems to matter; a state coined by Hungarian-American psychologist Mihaly Csikszentmihalyi as "flow". In this flow state, we feel alert, strong, in effortless control, and most notably, passionate about life.

Someone who gardens may find themselves working in their yard for hours at a time, and then wonder where the time has gone. Many crafters or home-renovators can feel the same way, and people can lose themselves in reading or even conversing with a friend. When we are so absorbed into a moment that nothing else seems to matter, we find ourselves calm but also energized. We feel our best.

SHOJIN-RYORI-INSPIRED *GOMA-DOFU*

4 servings

When you want to make and eat something beautiful, this *shojin-ryori*-inspired *goma-dofu* is a beautiful addition to any *ichiju-sansai* meal. While not quite as time-consuming as the traditional recipe – which requires grinding your own white sesame seeds with a mortar and pestle – this dish can remind us of the value of simplicity and taking the time to make things at home rather than buying what's made in-store.

Ingredients
- 50g/1¾oz white sesame paste (neri-goma)
- 50g/1¾oz potato starch
- 1 tsp dashi powder
- 400ml/14fl oz/1¾ cups warm water
- pinch of salt
- wasabi and soy sauce to taste (optional)
- Rectangular pan: Use a small vessel that is at least an inch deep, and about 4.5in x 5.5in. You may choose to use a circular pan if you'd like; the tofu will just come out in a circular shape.

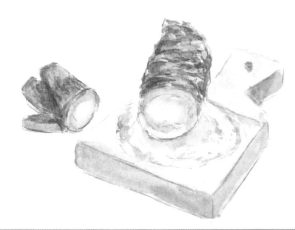

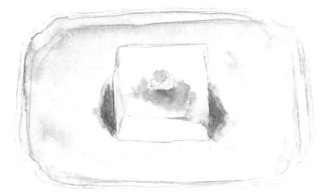

Instructions:

1. Dampen a flat rectangular pan with water so it is wet. Set aside.
2. In a medium pot, using chopsticks or a whisk mix the potato starch, dashi powder, and water until uniform.
3. Add the sesame paste and salt, and mix well.
4. Place the pot mixture over a medium-low heat and mix continuously. Once it begins to come together, lower the heat and continue mixing until sticky.
5. Pour and spread the mixture in the flat pan, and place the pan in an ice-water bath or fridge for an hour to cool.
6. Cut with a wet spoon or knife and serve with wasabi and soy sauce.

People do not just snap into a flow state; to reach it requires patience with ourselves, and a consistent reminder to take our time rather than feel rushed through the process.

By slowing down and allowing ourselves to focus, we eventually become fully immersed, which leads to joy for the moment rather than being distracted by other thoughts. Time-consuming activities are not bad for us; choose the right ones, and they can help us feel more awake and at peace.

It's easy to dismiss slowness as dull, but the adrenaline-chasing mindset is unsustainable and can cause us to lose sight of the larger meaning behind our actions, which can eventually lead to chronic anxiety and suffering – a condition that is often colloquially referred to as "hurry sickness".[43] It's not just the emotional consequences, such as difficulty concentrating, uncontrollable irritability, or feelings of inadequacy, but a chronic sense of feeling rushed can lead to physical symptoms such as trouble sleeping, headaches, high blood pressure, and migraines. Even if we are doing work that we love, surrounded by people we care about, a life that doesn't allow time for rest is a life we learn to resent.

It is important to note that slowing down is not necessarily about distracting ourselves or simply filling our time with something else to do. Oftentimes people turn to activities like scrolling through social media or watching Netflix during their breaks, but more often than not these activities do not make us feel more refreshed or open-minded to different possibilities – they still wire us to think and move fast. Instead we should think of rest as a way to allow not just our body but our mind to move slower. I will explain how to best encourage this in the following lessons.

As an aside, I think it is worthwhile to mention that while there are many activities we can turn to for slowing down, I will primarily advocate for engaging with activities that are of non-digital means. It can be difficult to notice the details when we are interacting with mediums designed for entertainment and instant gratification, such as social media or video games, applications that are designed with efficiency, speed, and fast-moving content at their forefront. While it is not impossible to find helpful digital means when we are looking to slow our brains down and find details worth paying attention to, the physical world tends to be much more conducive to this mindset.

"Making time for slowness allows us to re-examine our values and rearrange our priorities."

Slowness may cause some personal discomfort, for it does not always feel natural to embrace taking our time when it seemingly accomplishes less, but building a quality and meaningful life, like all things, is best accomplished when we move in moderation. Making time for slowness allows us to re-examine our values and rearrange our priorities so we have breathing room in our lives for more creativity, risk, and fun. So when you find yourself moving too fast, don't be afraid to pause, take a breath, and slow down a bit.

Lesson 10: Slow down

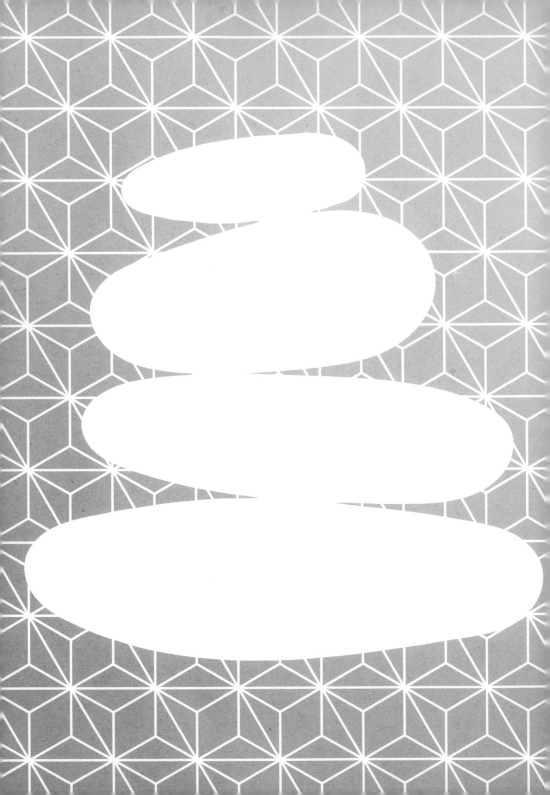

LESSON 11:

BE CURIOUS

It is easy to verbalize and understand the importance of slowing down, but where most people struggle is going from slowing down to entering that state of total immersion and mindfulness. We easily become interrupted by other thoughts floating around in our mind, by tempting distractions in our vicinity, or visual reminders of something else we should or could be working on. It is even more frustrating when you are trying so hard to focus and you find your mind constantly wandering. Sometimes we try to force ourselves into focus – why can't our brain just obediently do one thing at a time? – but this often just leads to more frustration, and our mind continues to scatter and race. This is known as the paradox of control: the more you try to control something, the harder it becomes to control.

This is how attempting to write this book felt: like trying to grab at falling flower petals, the more desperately I tried to snatch them, the more quickly they whooshed out of reach. But luckily, I had found a helpful teacher who helped me realize that sometimes if you just let things be, you can find the flower petal naturally floats down into your hand. Her example helped me discover how to overcome my self-prophesying frustrations. Who was my teacher? My three-year-old cousin.

If you have kids, or otherwise have watched a child entertain themselves before, you'll notice that children do not worry about why they are doing something, if they are doing it exactly right, or whether it is even useful to their life. I spent one summer watching my cousin pick up beach sand and mold it into little balls, or hop on the swings and pretend the wind rushing through her hair was how flying would feel. She would sit and observe ants for hours, and would experiment with dropping sugar cubes around their nest just because she wanted to see what would happen. She would pull out grass, sniff it, and then hand it to me like it was the most interesting thing you could share with someone.

Since then, whenever I found myself stuck with writing, before jumping in I would first take a moment to imagine talking to my three-year-old cousin instead. I told her how I was feeling and what I was struggling with, and then asked for advice on what she thought would be interesting for people to read about. I'd imagine she'd say something silly and perhaps a bit eccentric in response, and then move on with her day. I reminded myself that I could do the same if I wanted. Try something out, see what happens, and figure out what to do from there.

Instead of trying to force yourself into concentration, what can be helpful instead is to first embody a child-like mindset of playfulness. Because when you were a child, how would you approach an activity? You probably wouldn't be too concerned with the outcome, and you most likely wouldn't be concerned with achieving mastery. Instead, playfulness helps us let go of our anxieties and instead lean into curiosity, which is often the foundation of concentration. While it is difficult to pay attention to activities that stress or bore us, activities that we are curious about can quickly draw us in and captivate us for long periods of time.

"Playfulness helps us let go of our anxieties and instead lean into curiosity."

The value of embodying a playful and curious mindset doesn't just apply to work or the things we have to do; we can apply it to the activities we do for relaxation as well. For example, if you are interested in art, painting may be a suitable activity for decompressing. Let's say you take this desire to paint to find rest from work, but maybe you find yourself unable to enjoy painting because you are too anxious about an upcoming project deadline. You understand that you must slow down and do something else so you do not burn out from work, but you're too anxious to actually use the activity to calm your mind. Painting starts to feel like procrastination rather than a useful tool for de-stressing.

Instead of letting yourself grow frustrated because you are unable to enjoy your slowing-down activity, take that time to begin asking yourself questions. What does the paper feel like? How about the paint? In what way does the paintbrush tip interact with the paper, and how might that change if you used a different brush? What do the colors look like, and how do they blend together? What else might a child ask? What might a child do instead?

What you may notice is that the voice in your head that was distracted with other thoughts, is beginning to be replaced with one that is more present with what you're currently working on. You may notice that you begin to view your world a little differently, through a slightly different lens than you had before. You may start to become more curious about the little things that you couldn't see when you were moving too fast, and more deeply interested in what is facing you at present.

We can practice this exercise with anything that we like to do to relax. If you enjoy cooking, try asking yourself questions about the ingredients you're working with – what does it feel like? How does it smell? How does it taste raw, and how does the texture and flavor change after you cook it? If you enjoy listening to music, try asking questions about the beat, the way the melody makes you feel, what it reminds you of, or what the lyrics of the song mean to you. Be curious, ask questions, and you may find yourself slowing down.

Often this attention to detail manifests itself as an idea commonly referred to as *kodawari* in Japanese. It is about paying attention to the little details and being thoughtful about the smallest of things. In painting it can be caring about the texture of a piece of paper, the shape of a paintbrush's handle, or the consistency of the paint that you might be working with. In cooking it may be about the quality of the ingredients or the knife's edge; in music it may be the quality of your speakers or the environment in which you listen to it.

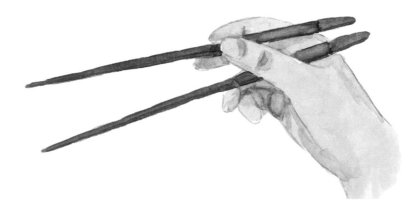

In most contexts *kodawari* is interpreted as the relentless pursuit of perfection, which may seem at odds with the principle of curiosity and slowing down. But upon closer inspection of the nuance behind the word, it becomes much clearer that *kodawari* is not the same as perfectionism, and when harnessed correctly it can be used to better the spirit of our wellbeing and expand our bandwidth for life.

Kodawari is better understood as a pursuit of perfection that acknowledges it is not possible to achieve, but it is nonetheless worth trying to get as close to it as possible. It's often a journey that starts off with noticing a very small detail about something in our environment – maybe the texture of a fabric doesn't feel quite right, the shape of a chair isn't as comfortable as it could be, or the sweetness of a fruit is not fully enhanced to its potential – and a curiosity is sparked within the individual that perhaps they can do something to make it better somehow.

Thus experimentation begins. It is the spirit of a *shokunin* – or artisan – that's ignited at this point, an internal drive that is born from an interest in something that seems almost insignificantly small. While some may perceive this as obsession, there is an aspect of altruism in the *shokunin* spirit; that any effort to improve an object doesn't need extensive justification other than that it will be more useful to the user and more respectful of the materials it is built with. It is an excellence-seeking perfectionism rather than a failure-avoiding perfectionism, which allows us to see our role and our contributions as part of a much bigger system, a recognition in which we find vitality.

This spirit of Japanese craftsmanship implies experimentation and a process of trial and error. It's about being open to what could or could not happen, which allows one to focus on the present condition, rather than becoming too concerned about the outcome of an experiment. In fact, skilled artisans understand that they can't be distracted by concerns. Each work session they need to pay their full undivided attention to the details of which tools and materials are being manipulated, the environment they are working in, and how to approach their craft. Some individuals spend a lifetime getting to know their chosen materials – one famous Japanese pottery artisan named Soetsu Yanagi described a need to "listen to" your materials, and understand their unique condition each time, as it can change from day to day, or even by the hour.[44] If the material is too stubborn to bend to the artisan's wishes, it is the responsibility of the artisan to notice, take a step back, and respect the craft: Okay, how can we approach it differently this time.

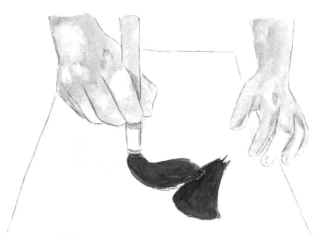

CALMING TRADITIONAL MATCHA

1 serving

Making your own matcha tea using a tea whisk may seem tedious at times, but the act of doing things properly allows us to slow down and become more thoughtful with the small details. We learn to notice that the process of making something can bring enjoyment that is much more meaningful to us. Enjoy with some small cookies or on its own, take deep breaths and let yourself sink into the joy of drinking tea.

Ingredients
- 2g matcha powder
- 60ml/2fl oz/¼ cup water

Essential Tools
- tea whisk
- hand sifter
- large ceramic mug or bowl

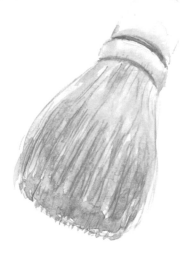

Instructions

1. Sift matcha powder into a large ceramic cup or small bowl to ensure there are no clumps.
2. Boil water and bring down to around 80°C/176°F, or let it cool for about 3–4 minutes.
3. Pour the water into the powder and quickly whisk the tea up and down, following the shape of an "M" as you do so.
4. Once well mixed and slightly foamy, enjoy!

"Passion is the result of slowing down and giving ourselves the bandwidth to question, explore, and experiment."

It is a common misconception that curious and passionate people like *shokunins* are born innately curious and passionate. Passion is the result of slowing down and giving ourselves the bandwidth to question, explore, and experiment, which gives us the energy to become passionate about something. We can't find this passion when we are stressed, distracted, or moving too quickly in life – it can only be found when we are slowing down and being mindful of the details in our present environment.

Mindfulness-based practices have been shown to physically change areas in our brains that are related to our emotions and behavior,[45] and research has shown that the practice is significantly effective at helping to reduce anxiety and depression symptoms in individuals, whether they suffer from severe or mild symptoms.[46] One study even showed it to reduce blood pressure in adults diagnosed with prehypertension,[47] suggesting that mindfulness could even help reduce stress on our bodies, and lower the risk for heart disease. It's amazing how closely interrelated our minds can be to our physical health.

Many people believe mindfulness is difficult to embody, but there is no need to be intimidated by it. It is really just the practice of stepping out of your autopilot mode and spending some time focusing on what your senses are telling you. What do you see? What do you feel? Are there any sensations that you hadn't noticed before? When we decide to focus on and immerse ourselves in activities that we inherently enjoy and are curious about, asking subtle questions about the medium at hand and then answering them, it can often be enough to quiet the voice in our head of distractions.

Curiosity also serves the additional benefit of keeping us resilient, another key to long-term sustainability and preventing ourselves from emotional burnout. When I was younger, I used to think that resilience just wasn't a skill I had; I've always considered myself to be on the more sensitive end (in other words, I easily cry), and I viewed resilience and feeling my feelings as being mutually exclusive.

When we speak about resilience in western contexts, most people believe it is about the endurance of hardship without emotion. We see a resilient person as someone who is easily able to laugh something off, or is able to be emotionally unbothered by rejection or failure. But I don't quite think that anymore – much like how courage is not the absence of fear, resilience is not the absence of a difficult emotion.

This is a particularly important mindset that is not spoken about often enough in the world of health. When people embark on their health journeys, what often happens is people set high-stakes expectations for themselves, overtax their bodies, and overburden their minds with the pressure of having to succeed, and that they must be "resilient" throughout the experience. In reality, resilience is not an emotion, but is about the ability to take action despite emotional hardship. For me, this was key to my own health journey.

> "Much like how courage is not the absence of fear, resilience is not the absence of a difficult emotion."

When I was struggling with my weight, I had a habit of buying fried chicken from the convenience store on my way home from school. It was hot and crispy and came in a cute and colorful illustrated packet. I thought it was the most delicious thing. I discovered it by happenstance, but what first started out as a novelty became a daily occurrence, and I found that eating fried chicken after school became almost a ritual. Even when I wasn't hungry, I felt compelled to buy and eat it. When I noticed this, I panicked – is this becoming a pattern? Will this be another unhealthy habit that I won't be able to break?

At this time though, I was already done with emotionally beating myself up. I didn't want to feel guilty for eating fried foods, and

I wanted to treat myself with more kindness. A kinder version of myself would not get upset or feel ashamed for this, but they would also have my best interests in mind. They would want me to be healthy, but how? What might this kinder version of myself suggest instead?

Try being curious.

So I experimented a bit. I replaced my fried chicken with onigiri rice balls. I tried making it an event, where I would walk to a local park instead of straight back home to enjoy my snack. I eventually made the distance a bit longer, and found myself walking for 30 minutes before eating. I then replaced my walk with a 10-minute jog to save time. My jogs became 15 minutes, then 20 minutes. Then I found that if I exercised, I was no longer very tempted to eat. The ritual of eating fried chicken had lost its glow.

It was not a linear transition; I had days where I would hide in bed because I ate too much and was feeling really uncomfortable in my own skin. I'd avoid mirrors on other days, or choose to shut myself in my room. I sometimes cried. But these bouts of sadness never lasted too long, because I would always think about the kinder version of myself. They'd let me cry, but they'd get up from bed. They'd give me a hug, and then nudge me to get out of my room. It may not have been linear but changing my routine didn't feel tiring because the habit change was so emotionally low-stakes. I found myself thinking: Learning to be healthier can feel this way?

When people commit to stoicism during their health journey, it can end up feeling like a measure of your success, that feeling sad or dispirited because something didn't go as you planned is a sign that you are not capable of reaching your goals, but that is not what these emotions are telling you at all. Our emotions are there to provide important information about what's going on around us, hints as to what's working and not working, but it doesn't speak to our capability.

Staying curious can help us remind ourselves of this truth and to accept our feelings without judging them, which can lift the emotional pressure from ourselves. We feel less worn down. We feel lighter. When I need to remember that, I like to turn to a few of my favorite Japanese proverbs that have helped me reconsider what resilience looks like:

1. **Even monkeys fall from trees** (猿も木から落ちる)

    Everyone makes mistakes. This is a fact of life. Professionals, experts, mentors, and leaders – even the most qualified people in their fields and positions will mess up on occasion.

    And if they're allowed to make mistakes, you are, too. Falling may hurt, and it might be a bit embarrassing, but it doesn't define your self-worth. Try to embrace it for what you can learn from it. A monkey that falls out of the tree isn't doomed to stay on the ground forever.

2. **Flexibility conquers rigid strength**
    (柔能く剛を制す)

    Stubbornness may be more intimidating, but flexibility can be much more powerful in the end. Instead of resisting, bending to what we can't control can prevent us from breaking. If we want to find a sustainable path, we have to notice that there's a time for fighting and a time for letting go. We can be flexible with what comes our way.

    We may even discover a better path.

3. Fall down seven, stand up eight (七転八起)

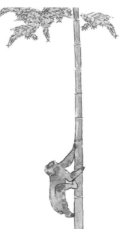

Sometimes we mess up. We fall. That's okay. We have permission to sit and cry, give ourselves some recovery time, and seek some support and consolation from others. There's no rush – the most important thing is that you get back up eventually, whenever and however makes sense for you. You don't need to tamp down your feelings or put a positive spin on everything that comes your way. Resilience can mean crying, processing your sadness, bending to the forces that threaten to knock you over, and then, eventually, choosing to climb back up the tree. That's demonstrating resilience.

Whether you are embarking on a new health journey, trying to pick up a new skill or hobby, looking to step up your career, or otherwise self-improve in another manner, first allow yourself to embody a curious, almost playful, mindset. This mindset can help us overcome the paradox of control, become more concentrated in our work and hobbies, and weather failure when we inevitably face it. You will find that you are less likely to psyche yourself out of challenges and activities that interest you and easing the emotional pressure can make you feel more energized. Instead of feeling anxious, we find ourselves calmer and more controlled, more willing to slow down and foster our passions. Seeing the world through new eyes may seem like an act only reserved for young children, but we can nurture our focus and attention with just a little effort: all it takes is leaning into our curiosity.

Lesson 11: Be curious

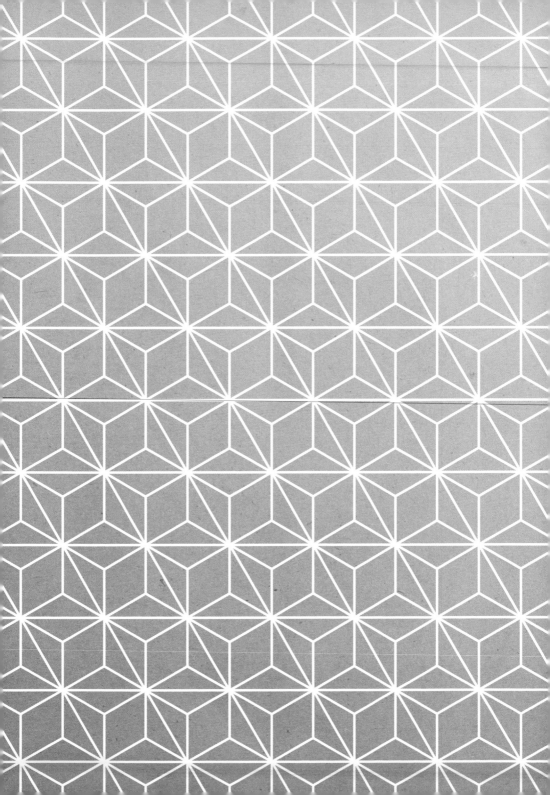

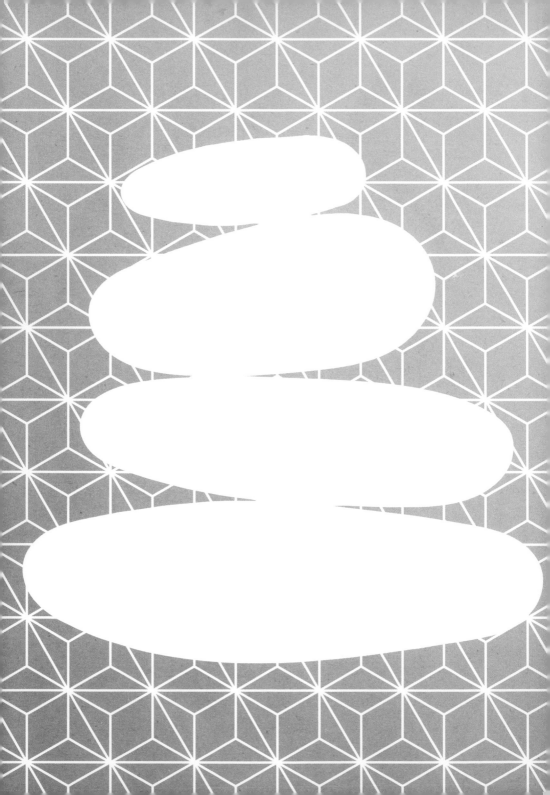

LESSON 12:
CARE FOR YOUR SURROUNDINGS

When understanding how to slow down, there is one more vital thing we should pay attention to: our surroundings. Creating a space that is conducive to rest does not just mean cozy pillows and warm lighting, but is about creating space that allows us to feel peace and calm.

What do you visualize when you think of rest? What kind of environment do you think it takes place in? If you were to ask a Japanese person, they would probably describe rest as a person leaning against a tree.

人: *person*

木: *tree*

休: *rest*

The Japanese character for rest is the combination of "person" and "tree". It's a universal image, the person leaning against the tree to rest - a representation of rest as not simply sleep or the absence of work, but about being in a safe place, somewhere we can feel peace.

Recent work-from-home set-ups have tempted many of us to blend our environments – to eat where we work or work where we sleep – but this merge of environments has made places that are traditionally designed for rest into spaces that aren't conducive to finding peace. When we see our work laptop we are reminded of our unread emails, and when we see the stack of mail in the corner we are reminded of our unpaid bills. It doesn't matter if there is urgency to these responsibilities or not, but their presence can make simple events that should be relaxing – such as enjoying a meal at the kitchen table – something quite difficult to enjoy.

The idea that the things in our vicinity consciously or unconsciously influence us may not be new to us. Restaurants may decorate their walls with plant life to solidify their farm-to-table branding, or retail

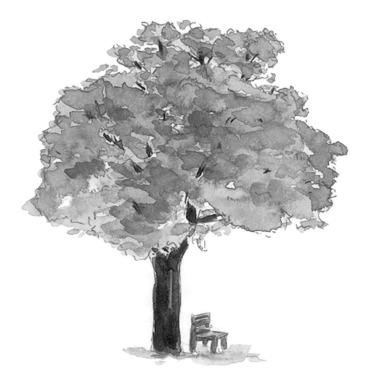

stores may design their floors with marble to make the customer feel important and wealthy. Teachers often put up motivational posters in the classroom to encourage students to be more confident, hard-working, or kind to others, and we remind ourselves of the love in our lives when we put up photos of our family and friends.

While we are often focused on what we can add to our rooms and spaces to make them more inspiring, comfortable, or peaceful, we should also pay attention to what we need to remove from our surroundings to make them less stressful, tense, or anxiety-inducing. This doesn't mean we need to clear an entire room for a home office or dining room – unfortunately, we don't always have the means or space to do so – but we should be mindful of clearing away unopened mail from the kitchen table when we eat or putting away our laptop and work papers when we go to sleep. Simple things with an immediate impact.

Japanese imagery of rest showed me that the rest isn't found in a vacuum, that we can't just close our eyes and put in our earplugs if we want to feel rested. Instead of trying to just block them out, what we really need is to feel safe from the distractions of life: we need to be under our tree.

Minimalism, a popular lifestyle movement inspired by Japanese traditional Zen Buddhism, reflects this importance of intentionally living with only the things we need to bring us a sense of peace and safety. Central to its belief is that having less is doing more, and that when examined closely most things in our life can be removed to create space.

If you are unfamiliar with Japanese minimalism, it may be helpful to start off with the example of bedding. Unlike western beds, Japanese beds are traditionally laid on the floor, as thick mats called futons. Rather than leaving them out all day, they are folded and put away every morning to make more space in the room.

I used to think that this was very tedious. Why does one not leave it out during the day if they are just going to come back to it at night? Growing up I had been used to western beds, but every time I went back to Japan during the summer to visit my grandmother, she would make us put away the futon every morning and every

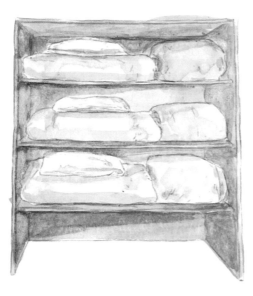

evening pull it out again to make our bed. Even as a child, it did not make much sense to me.

But I realized that when we forgot to put away the futons, there was a marked difference in how welcoming that room felt. Suddenly there was no space on the floor to play games, and we were stepping on and trampling over blankets and pillows with our feet. Everything became a mess, and the room felt chaotic. I would sometimes find myself wishing that my grandmother had forced us to put away our futons rather than leave my siblings and I to our own devices.

Having fewer things around us can make life a lot less stressful. But it is important to understand that at its core, this minimalism is not simply about reducing our belongings, it's about examining a lifestyle that is better for us when we have less in it. Simply having less stuff doesn't bring us joy, but the absence of things that bring us chaos can make us calmer and more content. It's about only having what's necessary out in your vicinity, and everything else is either put away or let go of.

"It's not simply about reducing our belongings, it's about examining a lifestyle that is better for us when we have less in it."

Living in an organized environment doesn't just make us feel more at peace but can visibly impact the way our brains work. A 2011 study using fMRI brain scanning technology showed that visual disorganization and clutter literally changes the way our brains work, making it harder for participants to focus and process information.[48] Yet when these same participants were moved to organized spaces, their productivity significantly improved. Visual clutter can also negatively impact our working memory,[49] and an overwhelm of stuff can also make us inclined to eat more unhealthy food than we might otherwise eat.[50] We begin to think through the filter of stress, rather than need.

The value of Japanese minimalism doesn't necessarily mean that we all should be replacing our western beds with Japanese futons. It is simply to recognize that tidiness is not merely tedious, and that being mindful of having less stuff in our immediate vicinity carries real value to our health and wellbeing. This may mean letting go of some things, or this may just mean getting into the habit of putting things away. It can be either, as long as we are mindful of removing things that bring us chaos, so we feel calmer and more content in the present moment.

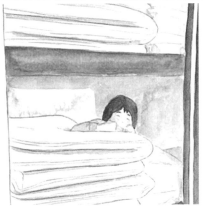

Most Japanese children learn the importance of taking care of the spaces they occupy early on in their life through the school system. In Japanese public schools and many private schools, there are no janitorial or cleaning staff to pick up after the daily mess left behind by students and teachers. When janitorial staff are employed, they tend to only be responsible for repairs or deep-cleaning that students may not be capable of doing on their own. In principle, everyone is expected to clean up after themselves.

Students will be as young as first graders (ages 6-7) when they are first given the responsibility of cleaning. For about 20 minutes each day, students are handed brooms, rags, and brushes, and are assigned to either the classrooms, hallways, bathrooms, or locker rooms to tidy up. While it may seem improbable that young students would take such a daily chore seriously, students quickly pick up on how they will be spending their school days in clutter and grime if they don't. Everyone has a part to play.

In this way, individuals become much more attuned to their environment and how it affects their school-life experience, and build the skills to maintain their spaces and keep it organized. Athletes are keen to keep basketball courts properly swept, and lab students are attentive to keeping their workspaces organized and clean. Students keep their desk and common spaces clean, because if they don't do it themselves, nobody else will.

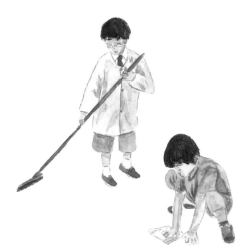

Of course keeping tidy may feel like a chore at times, but it should be to the same extent that brushing your teeth may feel like a chore - necessary, but mostly intuitive and natural to the daily routine. There is no need to conduct a whole cleaning overhaul of your home to integrate the art of tidiness into your lifestyle. In fact, instead of overwhelming yourself with an extreme lifestyle change, like everything we've been speaking about so far, the most effective thing to do is to start slowly and with moderation in mind.

If you're just a curious beginner, I like to say that the best way to get started with the habit of tidiness is to make your bed every morning. Just by making your bed, you'll begin to see what you have too much of and ways to tidy and set up a space that is central to the way you begin and end all of your days. Do you have too many pillows? Are there crumbs in your bed? Making the bed should only take 10 to 20 seconds at most, but it's enough to help us build into our routine the habit of tending to our spaces and reflecting on how they impact our emotional wellbeing. At the very least, it always feels nice to crawl into a ready-made bed at the end of the day.

"The most effective thing to do is start slowly and with moderation in mind."

Creating a space that is conducive to rest does not have to be about dedicating a whole room to one function, or following minimalist ideals of getting rid of everything unnecessary to a tee, but it is about being mindful of our surroundings, and taking care of them in a way that allows us to enjoy a more calm mindset. Small changes in our environment can be enough to make a meaningful impact to our ability to slow down.

Lesson 12: Care for your surroundings

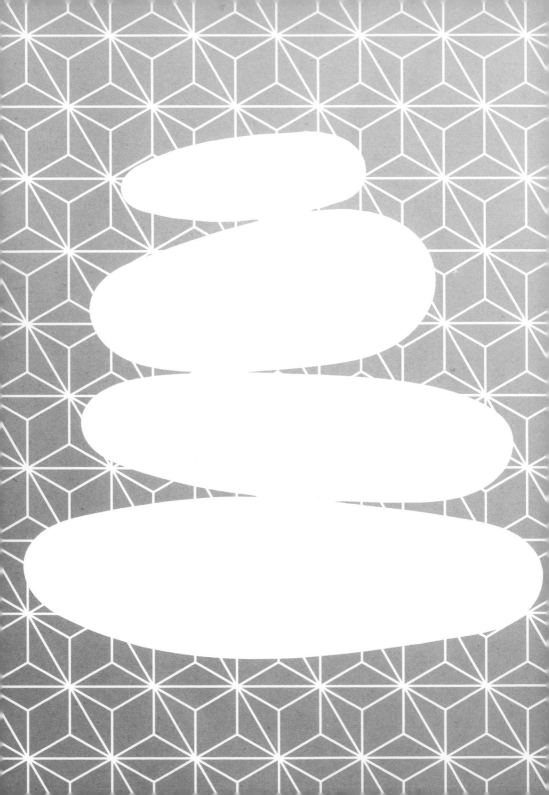

LESSON 13:
LEAN INTO
SPIRITUALITY

The final lesson to rest is about what we can do when we feel as though we are lost, and are not really sure where to begin when it comes to slowing down. Sometimes the stresses in our life are not things that are easily put away, and we need support from some other place to find the bandwidth to slow down. What I have found most helpful in times like these, when it feels like I don't have many options, is tuning into my spirituality.

If you consider yourself religious, you may understand what I am talking about. Religion offers individuals a sense of peace and directed guidance in an otherwise big world full of unknowns. If you do not consider yourself religious or spiritual, you may be wary of what it means to put belief in the intangible. I understand it is not easy to trust that which can't be proven, and I am not going to convince you of a certain belief or value system. Instead I will offer an insight on spirituality that can help us find relief and calm, without having to think too deeply about it.

Let me start with a question that you may be thinking right now: "Are Japanese people religious?"

It's a question that I often get and have struggled to answer with defining clarity.

I was raised without clearly knowing what religion my family followed, but with the understanding that there probably was a belief we did follow – I engaged frequently in prayer, especially if there was a holiday or I was visiting an old family home, and I grew up in a place where there were hundreds of shrines across the city. But I was never encouraged to call myself religious.

Officially there are two main belief systems in the country, Buddhism and Shintoism. There are many large Buddhist temples and Shinto shrines scattered throughout the country, and even small neighborhoods usually have their modest local shrine. As of 2016, there are approximately 80,000 Buddhist shrines and Shinto temples respectively in Japan.[51] For context, there are about 40,000 church buildings in the UK.[52]

During national holidays such as New Year's or Obon, an annual Japanese Buddhist event to honor one's ancestors, people will often visit their family graves to pay their respects, and at other times many will regularly visit temples and shrines to pray. It is not uncommon for a household to carry a small Buddhist altar called a *butsudan* in the home for praying as well.

With all these practices in place, on the surface it would seem Japan is steeped in religion, but many people do not call themselves religious. According to a survey conducted in 2019, about 81 per cent of respondents said that they have never participated in a specific religious group.[53] In a separate national survey conducted in 2013, about 72 per cent of Japanese adults answered that they did not identify as religious.[54] Yet the most curious thing is when that same group of adults were asked whether they thought it was important to have a religious spirit, 66 per cent of the respondents had answered that it was important.

So why does it feel odd to identify as Buddhist or as a practitioner of Shintoism for many people, even though they engage in these practices? Do these practices not make one religious?

Many Japanese people hold a strong respect for forces beyond their understanding, and have a tradition of praying to their ancestors or praying to forces of nature, but they see these acts as cultural or personal values, rather than a piety to any one institution's causes. Instead of rules of what to do or not do, there is a pervading notion that Buddhism and Shintoism aren't the kinds of religions that have a supreme god, but are beliefs guided by spirits who act more like teachers.

In this sense, this belief allows praying to seem a bit more casual, and perhaps closer to the self. Teachers are to be respected, but they aren't necessarily meant to be worshiped. It may also account for why there are so many shrines and temples in Japan, because places of spiritual significance are thought to be accessible to the average person and not to be made out of reach. You can find places of worship near train stations, by the park, near hiking trails, and on top of rocks by the beach shore. They're not always impressive or particularly grand, but you're bound to come across one or two on your way home from work whether you live in a large city like Tokyo, or in a small rural town.

No matter who you are or where you live, there are times in our lives when we do not have control over the outcome of something, and we may feel a bit stressed or worried by this prospect. This is not something that should go unaddressed, for a prolonged sense of lack of autonomy can lead to mental health concerns like anxiety, depression, and low self-esteem. While many of us have maybe been told to just let it go or not worry about it, because what else is there to do, sometimes knowing that there is nothing we can do is not enough to let our minds feel at ease.

This is where I believe spirituality can lend a hand in supporting our needs.

WARABI-MOCHI

2 servings

On Japanese Buddhist altars people will often place *osonae* or food offerings, for their ancestors to enjoy with them. They frequently bring fresh seasonal fruit or vegan desserts, and will avoid foods that can spoil quickly or have meat as these are thought to dirty the altar. Rather than buy something specifically for the sake of offering, people will often choose to share what they are already enjoying at home – it doesn't necessarily have to be expensive or fancy, as long as it is shared with gratitude. *Warabi-mochi* is a simple yet delicious dessert that can easily be placed at an altar, and is one I hope you can enjoy and share with someone you'd like to pay respects to.

Ingredients
- 2 tbsp potato starch
- 1½ tbsp sugar
- 100ml/3½fl oz/scant ½ cup water
- 1 tbsp kinako powder
- kuromitsu (black sugar syrup) to taste

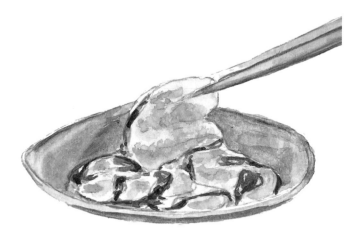

Instructions

1. Mix potato starch, sugar, and water in a microwave-safe bowl.
2. Microwave for 30 seconds on low.
3. Mix with wet chopsticks.
4. Repeat microwaving and mixing process 3 to 4 times until mixture becomes translucent. Set aside to cool.
5. Cover a large plate with kinako powder and place mixture onto the plate. Generously coat the mixture in the kinako powder.
6. Cut the warabi-mochi with a knife or spoon into bite-size squares.
7. Serve with kuromitsu and enjoy!

Spirituality may not directly lend autonomy, but it can at least increase our sense of security, and that is enough to improve our wellbeing and health. A study published in 2012 showed that people who responded that religion or spirituality was highly important to them were 76 per cent less likely to experience an episode of major depression[55] – curiously, their religious attendance or belief system had no significant impact on their likelihood of depression. Similarly, a 2008 meta-analytic review of 115 articles that studied the relationships between religion or spirituality and adolescent substance use, depression, and anxiety, found that 92 per cent of the studies observed a positive correlation between spirituality and better mental health. [56]

The Japanese model for spirituality shows that you do not need to be religious or identify with a specific religious organization to be spiritual, and that your beliefs surrounding God are not as important as your sense of faith in the intangible. Praying is compatible with the busy and modern lifestyle, and does not require a formal or structured effort. We can be spiritual in our everyday lives – on the way home from work or school, at a small butsudan altar inside the home, or simply before bed at night.

You don't need to be Buddhist to create a spiritual space in your home. If you are interested in learning how to create your own home altar, or a space similar to a butsudan, what you first need is a cleared-out designated area in a room where you can find some peace and quiet. Many people will choose an area close to a window or where there is ample natural lighting, so when they pray they feel more connected to nature. It doesn't need to be a large space, but make sure it is enough to fit a seat and desk.

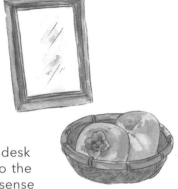

I recommend setting up a floor desk if possible, so you can be close to the ground. This can help give us a sense of stability and calm, as it narrows our peripheral vision and can help us focus on what is close to us rather than become distracted by other things in the room. Situating ourselves on the floor also makes sure that we are located physically below the altar, a sign of respect and attentiveness. However, it is more important that you feel comfortable and relaxed, and if sitting on the floor is uncomfortable for you it is perfectly fine to set up a chair and table; just make sure that the table is level or slightly higher than the chair so you don't find yourself towering over your altar.

Once you have a floor desk, make sure you have a comfortable cushion or soft carpet to sit on. It is common to use a *zabuton* (a Japanese sitting cushion) or *zafu* (a Japanese traditional meditation cushion), but depending on your preference you may choose to use a chair pad, car seat cushion, or a floor chair that has a back to it for support. Let yourself prioritize comfort when selecting a suitable cushion.

What goes on the desk to set up your altar is entirely up to you. Oftentimes people will include photos of their ancestors if they felt close to them, or a family heirloom that is representative of their lineage. In a spiritual space it is also important to engage the senses, so it is common for someone to leave an incense holder and some matches for when they pray. While the original purpose of burning incense when praying is still debated, it is generally used to sanctify a space and evoke the presence of spirits. Candles are also a great alternative to incense; something that can engage our senses and calm us.

And when you feel so inclined, you can dim the room, sit down by your altar, light the incense, close your eyes, and take a bit of time to pray. It's common for someone to pray for safety before traveling, or before a big event like an interview or exam. People also pray when they are going through hardship, or if they are looking for guidance on a major decision. Sometimes people simply pray in the morning before going to work, and will share a brief prayer before going to sleep at night. For extra luck, you can leave an *osonae* or food offering, something to show gratitude for your ancestors' presence.

Spirituality is also helpful to us because it offers us a practice of patience. Instead of stressing or panicking over what is outside of our control, we become more tolerant of uncertainty, and nudge ourselves to become more patient with the process. This is not the same thing as complacency, but it means to accept what is true in a moment, do what we can, and then find distance from our worries and anxieties. A study conducted in 2007 found that participants who were rated as more patient tended to experience less depression and fewer negative emotions,[57] and a separate study conducted in 2012 came to a similar conclusion:[58] that those who are patient with others tend to be less depressed, and more hopeful and satisfied with their own lives. When we can find acceptance, we can find more peace.

In Zen Buddhism, patience is often thought of as an act of compassion toward the self. It's quite easy to get wrapped up in frustration, but when we turn inwards it helps us move from a place of identifying by that frustration – I am a frustrated person – to simply identifying it as something we are experiencing – I am feeling frustration. This perspective shift can help us reflect that our emotions are not something we necessarily have to hold on to, but something that we may let go of.

"By learning to accept that which is true in a moment and notice what is out of our control, we can give ourselves more peace with the present."

There is a technique known as "Leaves on a Stream" created by Dr Russell Harris, that is often used in acceptance and commitment therapy, to help bring peace to the mind. One is asked to visualize themselves sitting beside a slow-moving stream, and to watch leaves float by on it. As they notice their inner voice, on each leaf they place their thoughts and feelings and watch them float away. The purpose of this exercise is not to make the thoughts disappear or force them out of our mind, but merely bring a small pause to the voice in our heads, and to recognize and become patient with what we may be thinking or feeling. The leaves move at their own pace and sometimes may get stuck somewhere, but eventually they move on with time.

By learning to accept that which is true in a moment and notice what is out of our control, we can give ourselves more peace with the present. Having faith in the intangible does not mean we grow complacent or that we must worship any sort of god if we don't wish to. Instead spirituality is simply showing compassion toward ourselves by becoming more patient with our reality and our feelings, and being able to see our world through a grander perspective.

Finally, spirituality also offers us a space to practice gratitude, a practice that has been shown to correlate with less depression, more motivation, and a more positive mental outlook overall.[59] An ethnographic study published in 2020 on Japanese elderly living in Osaka, all individuals in their 80s and 90s, found that many of these individuals practiced a view of gratitude that allowed them to experience the present through a more positive, hopeful perspective.[60] The research described that the hope they were embodying was less of a triumphant or excited sense of hope, but one that felt quieter and more reflective of the past.

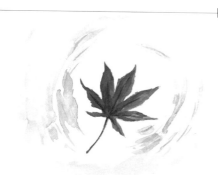

While many of the individuals in the study were hesitant to describe themselves as "happy", many of them responded that they were grateful for their lives. The participants recognized the difficulties and anxieties of growing older, but rather than cynicism, there was more acceptance of the present because they were recognizing that there was still much to be grateful for, and in turn, they felt a bit more peace and hope for the future.

It did not occur to me until much later in life, but when you pay close attention to the Japanese characters for "thank you", there is something a bit unexpected about the kanji.

有: **To have, possess**

難: **Difficulty, hardship**

有難う: **Thank you**

The Japanese characters for *arigatō*, thank you, are made up of the characters "to have" and "difficulty", and together they form the words "thank you". While many Japanese words come from the traditional Chinese alphabet, the words for thank you were thought to be developed by Buddhist linguists, based on their beliefs toward gratitude.

Arigatō means that good things in life are never obvious or a natural human right – there are so many things that can come in the way of something not happening or manifesting: wrong place, wrong

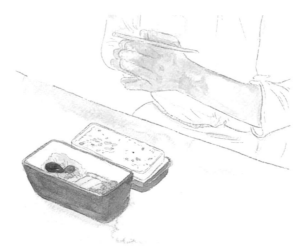

time, wrong person, wrong words – and consequently everything good that happens to us is a combination of many miracles. So being able to say thank you, even for the smallest of blessings, is not something we should take for granted. The ability to say thank you is, in fact, something to difficult to have.

What these characters recognize is that living is the world's greatest coincidence, all things considered with the universe's billions and billions of possibilities. To have restful sleep, nourishing meals, the ability to move, and sincere relationships – on the daily level we might find that they are obvious rights to possess, but upon closer inspection we realize that they are the outcomes of many odds, and that to have them is something to feel grateful for. To be spiritual is not necessarily about worship, but it can simply mean to be thankful to the intangible for bringing about these almost impossible odds.

If you already follow and practice spirituality, perhaps what I have shared already largely resonates in the context of your belief system. But even if you don't identify with a specific belief system, you don't need to overthink the act of praying or what spirituality means to you. It doesn't need to feel like an overwhelming or formal endeavor; being able to tune into an acceptance of the unknown and intangible can be a way for us to regain our sense of autonomy, practice patience with ourselves and our world, and embody a perspective that allows us to find gratitude in the peace of the everyday.

Lesson 13: Lean into spirituality

PILLAR 4:

SOCIALIZE

When we think about what we need to do to improve our health, many of us first think about making a change to our diet or getting more exercise, and some of us may get as far as thinking about sleeping earlier. It is evident to most of us that these lifestyle elements have the biggest impact on our health, and when successfully integrated they can be the most powerful preventative health measure we can undertake, but when neglected, these parts of our lifestyle can also contribute to our most fearsome health consequences.

So imagine how you would react if you went to the doctor to address high blood pressure, and instead of prescribing medication he prescribed you time with your loved ones. Imagine if he didn't

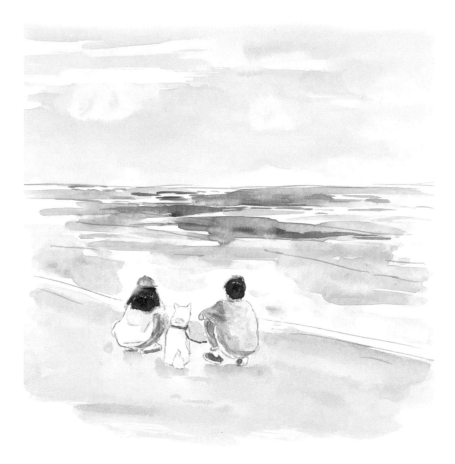

talk about eating more vegetables, getting more exercise, or why you need to be sleeping more. All he did was tell you to go spend more time with the people you love. We might be shocked, incredulous even.

Not many of us think about our family or friends when we think about our health, but the quality of our social relationships has an enormous impact on our physical and mental health. It is a crucial pillar to supporting our wellbeing. The director of the Harvard Study of Adult Development, Robert Waldinger, shared in a now-viral TED Talk about how his organization's lifetime study on US adults had found that the most important determinant for happiness and health in participants was the strength of their relationships with their family, friends, and community. [61]

Starting in 1938, the Harvard study followed the lives of two groups of men: the first group were sophomores attending Harvard College at the time, and the second group were those from Boston's poorest neighborhoods, individuals who were chosen because they came from disadvantaged backgrounds. Over their lifetime the researchers sent questionnaires, interviewed participants in-person, received medical records from their doctors, drew their blood, scanned their brains, and talked to their children. Consequently, the researchers found that wealth, fame, or hard work was not the main determinant of their health and happiness. It was the quality of their relationships.

Similar findings have been replicated elsewhere in the world as well; it is not just a phenomenon in the United States. A meta-analysis study conducted in 2015 uncovered that even when controlled for different world regions, loneliness and feelings of isolation increased the risk of early mortality, with some evidence that it may be as harmful to human health as obesity.[62] Being social is not just good for our mental health, it is one of the main factors impacting our physical health as well.

Japan's elderly are well-known for being active in their local communities well into their senior years. The Annual Report on the Ageing Society 2018 published by Japan's Cabinet Office found that about 70 per cent of people aged 60-69, and about half of those 70 and over, were engaged in some sort of social activity, whether this be working, volunteering, or taking lessons of some kind.[63] While we may not immediately think of social ties when considering community health, this active social participation among Japanese elderly may be one of the key factors to its relatively high longevity rates. An analysis on the health data of about 14,000 Japanese individuals aged 65 and older living in Aichi Prefecture in Japan, found that those who were married, exchanged contact with family members or friends, participated in community groups, or were working had a significantly lower risk of developing incident dementia than those who weren't.[64] Other studies conducted outside of Japan have also found that our sense of closeness with others is critical to our wellbeing,[65] and is one of the leading indicators of longevity and life satisfaction.[66] Our social life is critical to our health.

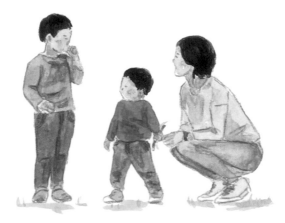

This is what I define as the fourth pillar to lifetime health: Socialization. To many of us it may seem obvious that to live a long and healthy life we need to eat well, get regular exercise, and sleep enough hours at night – our doctor tells us this, we were taught about it in health class, and we see ads for dieting and working out everywhere – but we cannot forget to look after the quality of our relationships either.

I would like to recognize that building meaningful relationships and deep connections with others can feel difficult for many people. It's a process that requires vulnerability and openness that not everyone is naturally equipped with, and that for some people being able to do this is an act of courage. Meeting new people and making close friends is not always an easy thing to do.

Personally, being overweight as a child made making friends difficult for me. But not in the way you might think – they say that kids are cruel, but I would say that one of the biggest hurdles to making close friends was not that other kids were mean to me, but that I had internalized a message that no one would want to be friends with someone overweight. So much so that I always knew what my teachers would write on my progress reports before opening the envelope: "This student is a pleasure to have in class but is a bit quiet and shy." I never saw it as a bad thing – I tried to protect myself by making my presence very small in social situations.

This strategy for social preservation had its drawbacks of course, the main one being that if I never put myself out there to get to know people, I couldn't make close friends. There was so much fear around being judged that I always waited for others to approach me, and when they did I made sure I was always pleasant and polite. Even the people I did get to know better I kept at arm's length. I reasoned it was fine and that friendships should feel like this, but I later realized that it was a very lonely experience.

It was my belief that popularity was the key to my happiness that led to my ironic tendency toward shyness so I wouldn't get judged. But I later learned that building a strong social network is not about being popular. It is not always enough to be outgoing or to have a large number of friends and close family, for we can feel lonely in a crowd as well. A strong social network is instead built on quality and genuine connections with others, but without the right guidance in trying to build these connections, our efforts can easily become time-consuming, energy-draining, and increasingly frustrating.

Many people think that as we grow older, we naturally become better at making friends because presumably our social skills are more refined, but loneliness is also very present among adults. A meta-analysis published in 2021 noted a trend of increasing loneliness in adults from 1976 until 2019.[67] Even if building meaningful connections wasn't difficult enough under normal circumstances, loneliness has only increased since the coronavirus pandemic in 2020. The Making Caring Common project by Harvard University conducted a survey in October of 2020 and found that 43 per cent of young adults reported increases in loneliness since the outbreak, and almost 36 per cent of all American adults felt "serious loneliness" overall.[68]

So how do we build meaningful relationships in life? Contrary to what I believed as a child, my appearance or ability to charm was not significant at all in my ability to build remarkable relationships. In fact, I found that it required much less skill than I had initially thought; rather it was about a willingness to challenge the narrative that no one would want to be friends with me. Regardless of whether you are extroverted or introverted, shy or bold, I believe that by practicing the following four lessons in our daily lives, each of us can naturally build sincere and remarkable relationships with others. Each lesson is designed to include acts that we can implement anywhere at virtually any time, and can be embodied by anyone of any background. So read on, for this is the final – and perhaps most influential – pillar to our wellbeing.

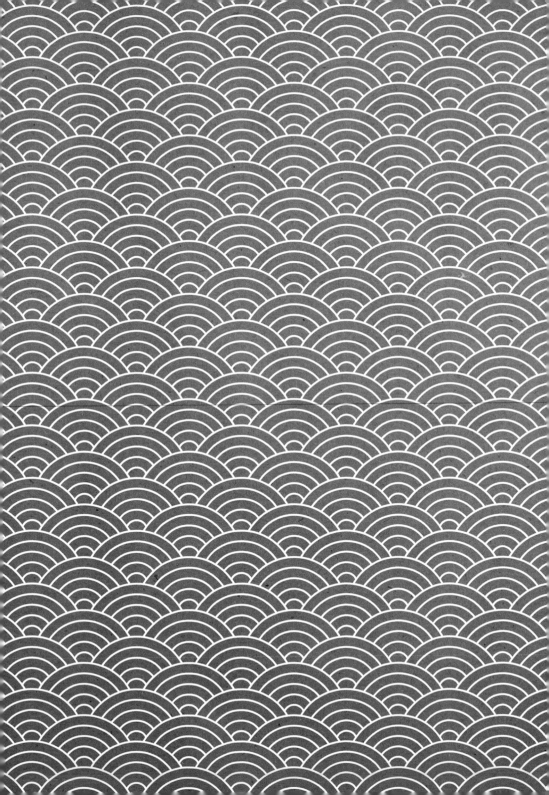

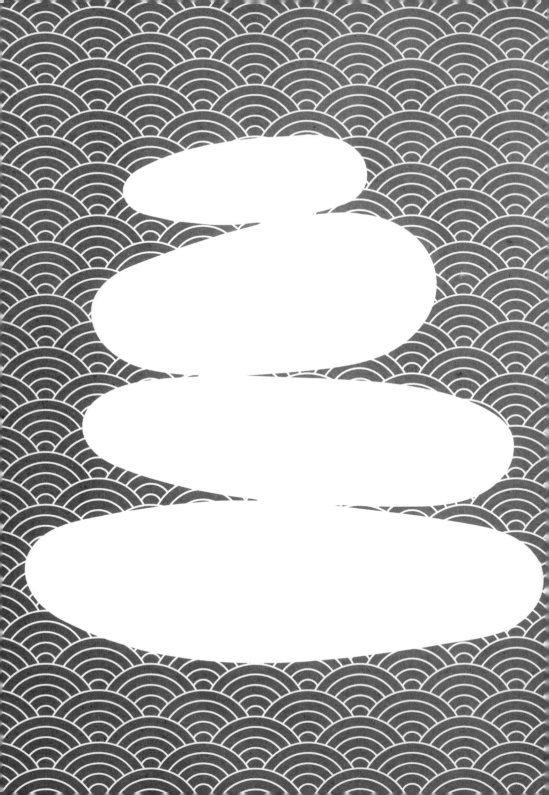

LESSON 14:

SAY HELLO AND LISTEN IN

How do we build deep and meaningful relationships? We must start at the very beginning and ask ourselves a much more simplified question: how do we make friends? This is where the more outgoing and confident of us have an easier time, but where the shy may already face difficulty. To make friends we must be sociable and likable, which is different from being popular, but to a degree, being liked by others is important to open the door to making friends.

Oftentimes when we want to make ourselves more likable, we believe that we need to change ourselves so others want to spend time with us. We may think we need to speak a different way, hold certain interests, be good at sports, or learn to be outgoing and funny in a crowd. We think we need to be charming or smart, and dress to impress. Yet we shouldn't change ourselves to fit in, for this disqualifies the ultimate goal of building meaningful and genuine connections. Not only should we not, but we don't have to change one thing about ourselves to be more likable. We can still be ourselves.

It's a lot easier to become more sociable and likable than we think. It doesn't require building upon and refining our communication and social skills, or learning to act and behave in any special way. The most fundamental thing we can do to be more likable is something anybody is capable of: say hello.

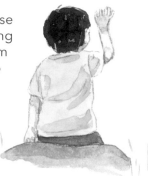

What kinds of greetings do you use every day? Do you say good morning or good evening? How about "I'm home!" or "Looking forward to working with you today." Who do you say greetings to, and in what context do you use them?

In Japanese society, greetings or *aisatsu* are used all the time. Beyond just hello or goodbye, it is common to say *ittekimasu* before leaving the house, or *okaeri nasai* to welcome someone else home. You may press your hands together and say *itadakimasu* before starting a meal, and when you are finished eating it is customary to say *gochisousama deshita* to thank the person who made your meal.

This practice is not just between family and close friends; they are encouraged at school, in the workplace, and in the public domain as well. If you enter a Japanese restaurant, someone may yell a cheery *irasshaimase* to welcome you in the door, or someone may bow and say *osewa ni narimasu* before entering a business meeting. When you leave a store you'll rarely leave in silence, as someone will most likely say *arigatō gozaimasu* or *mata yoroshiku onegaishimasu* to affirm that you're welcome back at any time.

Aisatsu are not just prevalent, but they're an important part of Japanese life. They're taught from a young age in schools and often reinforced in the home as part of the Japanese value system. Classrooms will often conduct a brief *chourei*, or morning greeting, before the school day begins, and companies will often host a similar morning stand-up to align everyone before starting work.

To value and practice *aisatsu* with others is believed to be a part of what makes one Japanese.

Aisatsu is a word with Zen Buddhist roots, composed of two characters which mean "to push" and "to close distance". Zen Buddhist linguists first understood *aisatsu* as a way to measure someone else's depth of enlightenment and open-mindedness, a back-and-forth act of asking many questions to understand someone else and read who they are. In this way, *aisatsu* was understood as putting yourself out there, or "pushing", to become closer with others. While this is the root of the word, over time *aisatsu* took on a much more casual role in Japanese society and simply became a tool to better connect with the people around us and invite them to become closer to us.

挨: *To push*

拶: *To close distance*

挨拶: *Aisatsu*

I won't forget the first person who really showed me the importance of Japanese *aisatsu*. It wasn't my parents or other family members, but in fact someone who was a stranger to me at the time. When I was living in New York my parents were still adamant that I receive a partial Japanese education, so they enrolled me in a Japanese Saturday school. Embarrassed by my lack of fluency compared to my classmates who had recently moved to New York from Japan, I quickly became known as the quiet, untalkative girl in the class. I was not outgoing to begin with, but the language barrier had really sealed my fate as someone who was unsociable, and in my early days at Saturday school I was quite friendless. That was, until one day a girl in my class decided to approach me with a simple *aisatsu: ohayo!*

TAKO-SAN WIENER

2 servings

I was a fairly shy person when I was young, but I found that bringing interesting and fun Japanese foods to school was a great way for me to talk to people. Cute and easy to make, *tako-san* wieners are popular bento box items in Japan to upgrade any normal lunch into one worth talking about with others. So if you're looking for a fun conversation starter with your friends or coworkers, look no further!

Ingredients
- 4 mini hot dogs
- 8 black sesame seeds for eyes

Essential tools
- Toothpicks

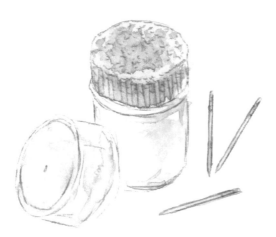

Instructions

1. Heat up a small pot of water to boil.
2. While waiting for the water to boil, using a knife carefully make an incision halfway up the hot dog. On the same end, perpendicular to your first cut, make another incision halfway up. You should end up with four "legs" on one end.
3. Do the same thing again on the same end, so you end up with eight evenly-sized "legs" on half of the hot dog.
4. Boil the hot dogs in the water for 30 seconds to a minute. The ends should expand so it looks like legs! Set aside and allow to cool.
5. Using a toothpick, gently poke the top end of the hot dog where you'd like the eyes to be, so there are small dents.
6. Gently place the black sesame seeds into the dents to create eyes.
7. Enjoy!

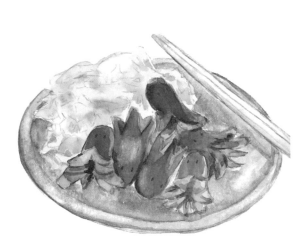

I was surprised by the gesture, but the girl had smiled and so I returned one back. It was the first time I really felt my presence being recognized by someone else. I didn't consider myself particularly social, but from that day on every time I saw her I would say a short greeting - *ohayo*! It was an easy, automatic gesture that made me feel better about being in the classroom. Eventually others started saying good morning to me, and I would return one to them. Over time the good mornings would extend into conversations, and slowly but surely, I found myself making a few friends.

"It's lovely to watch the way someone else's face lights up when you greet them."

Greetings may seem like such a trivial thing to reinforce in so many aspects of daily life, but I have come to understand that they serve a very important purpose. First, they validate another person's existence, which I believe is the foundation of human empathy and the bare minimum we must do to build meaningful relationships. Not only does it feel nice when someone we do not know well recognizes our presence, but doing that for someone else can possibly turn their whole day around. It's lovely to watch the way someone else's face lights up when you greet them.

Not just when you are trying to get to know someone, but consistently taking the time to notice others, is also important. It makes another person feel like they matter and evokes a sense of care and inclusion. Japanese teachers and school principals will often lead by example by standing in front of the school gates every morning to say *ohayo gozaimasu* ("good morning") to every student that enters. It sets the tone for the community, and a reliable greeting by a familiar face every morning can make someone feel seen.

Secondly, this can inspire conversation, a potential new beginning for friendship and community. Maybe they've noticed that you're good at math and can feel comfortable asking for your help with

186

something, or perhaps you realize that you both share a love for the same music group and make plans to see their next concert together.

My first day at college, after a long day of unpacking and sorting my things, I remember how quiet my room was. It was still early in the night, but I was jetlagged and decided that I wasn't ready to participate in the freshman parties just yet, so I went to the communal bathroom to get ready for bed. There was another girl there washing her face, also getting ready for bed, but I decided I wouldn't bother her and began brushing my teeth.

But then she noticed me, and her face still wet and soapy, she turned to me and gave me the biggest grin. "Hi, nice to meet you! I live in room 321; my name is Kayla." I tried to smile back but my mouth was full of toothpaste and I ended up dribbling something incoherent. Soapy face and drooly mouth, it was hardly a smooth introduction but we both laughed. We later discovered that we shared the same economics class and sat next to each other the entire semester. She is still one of my closest friends today.

It is much easier to make friends when that door to getting to know someone is already slightly open. We may never know where each new interaction may lead us.

Lastly, greetings open our hearts and minds to others. We may not know what someone else is thinking, or what their day had been like right before seeing us, but *aisatsu* allows us to think beyond ourselves and become genuinely interested in other people. Instead of being focused on how to make yourself interesting to others, it eases the pressure of having to make an impression, and instead creates a space for genuine curiosity.

"Meaningful relationships are ultimately built through meaningful conversations."

Aisatsu is an act that recognizes the people we meet in life will all be strangers to begin with, but that nobody needs to stay a stranger. Even if we feel as though there is distance created by age, gender, culture, or something less visible, by opening the door with a simple greeting, we can find ourselves growing closer with anyone around us.

While casual greetings open the door, meaningful relationships are ultimately built through meaningful conversations. This does not necessarily mean conversing about deep or serious topics, but it's about conversing in a genuine manner that is respectful of both people present – in simpler terms, it's about the art of listening.

Listening is not just about hearing the words and understanding what is being said, but skilled listeners are also able to use it as a way to communicate back. In Japanese culture, active listening practices – or the art of listening with all of your senses and showing attentiveness to the message being shared – are quite common in everyday conversations. If you were to mention this to someone who had been raised in Japan, they may tilt their head and question if this is true, but a foreigner living in Japan may understand. This is because active listening is not formally taught in Japan, but responsive body language and verbal cues are ingrained as a part of the cultural and conversational norm.

If you've ever watched a Japanese movie or witnessed a conversation in Japanese, you may have noticed an interesting relationship between the person listening and the person speaking. Usually when someone is listening intently you may expect them to be still and quiet, but in Japanese conversation, the person listening is often chiming in throughout the conversation, whether that be with words or movement. They may be nodding their head, throwing in a few "hai hai" or "un un" between sentences, or remarking with a *naruhodo* ("I see"). Seemingly pointless and usually instinctual than deliberate, these indications serve the same purpose: it's a form of communication back.

This communication is referred to as *aizuchi* (相槌) in Japanese: comments during a conversation that indicate to the speaker that the listener is paying attention. Literally translated, *aizuchi* means "mutual hammering" and refers to the back-and-forth communication a katana blacksmith master may have with their disciple. When teaching swordsmithing, a master and disciple take turns hitting the sword with a mallet, each fine-tuning to the other's marks and adjusting their pace to match in rhythm. The two must be present with each other, as something meaningful can be built only when both parties are in sync – like a conversation.

Aizuchi acknowledges that conversation requires participation from both sides to be meaningful, and so Japanese communication norms have evolved to incorporate nonverbal and visual cues as an important part of the dialogue. They are designed to make the other person feel at ease and assured that they are being understood, as the art of listening is not just listening, but being engaged and communicating this engagement.

"Something meaningful can be built only when both parties are in sync"

This is not to say that we should begin peppering our conversations with frequent head nods or interjectory sounds – especially if it is not culturally customary – but it is important to be aware of how we display and signal to others that we are actively present with them. What does your body language say? How are you showing responsiveness? Whether it be eye contact, touch, a smile, or the occasional affirming "I see" – by valuing the art of active listening, we are not only able to better understand what others are saying, but we are able to grow much closer with them.

The Japanese language recognizes there are two different kinds of listening- the first of which is simply hearing, where you can understand the words spoken by someone and repeat what they said back. This is characterized by the kanji "聞" (*kiku*), which includes the character for "ear".

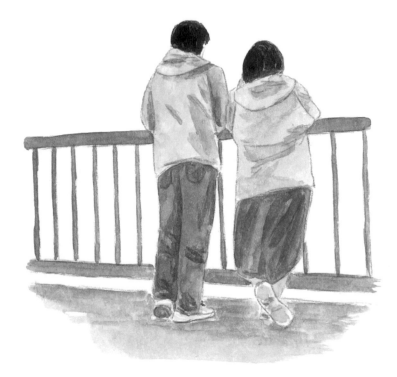

The second kind of listening is characterized by the kanji "聴く" (also *kiku*), but this one includes the character for heart: "心" (*kokoro*). Japanese uses this kanji when describing listening to music or listening to lectures, because it implies an instance where we're not just hearing things, but actively listening to seek understanding. In this form of listening, we are not simply hearing the sounds, but are actively engaged with what is being said.

Being sociable is not only reserved for the extroverted or forthcoming – the art of communication is accessible to everyone, at any level. We don't need to change ourselves to become likable, but it does require us to proactively engage with others around us – something as simple as a hello can do. Then once the doors to conversation are open, we can learn to facilitate meaningful interactions by honing our skills for active listening.

This is how to plant the seeds for meaningful relationships, and how we may enter or build communities that can serve us for years to come. We don't need to dress differently, talk differently, change our interests, or match the demeanor of those around us. By being authentically ourselves but open to possibility and exchange, we attract like-minded people and those we share values with, and eventually make the friends we work well together with. Every meaningful relationship is born from someplace quite simple.

We will have to be open to the possibility that not every interaction will end in a close relationship, but that's okay. Even "weak ties", or having a casual network of acquaintances, has been linked with positive social and emotional wellbeing.[69] There is also evidence that the more we have, the merrier: a study published in 2014 found that the more weak ties a person had in their social circle, whether that be the mailman or the neighborhood grocery clerk, the happier and more secure they felt in their community.[70] Casual relationships are not the same as disingenuous ones, and we should not dismiss the power of low-stakes relationships on our wellbeing.

Best case scenario, a hello leads somewhere beautiful, but even if it is not the beginning of a meaningful relationship, we don't lose anything by sharing a greeting – and at the very least we may end up making someone else's day. So try saying hello to someone and let yourself open up to them; you are equipped with the assurance that you only have something to gain from listening in.

Lesson 14: Say hello and listen in

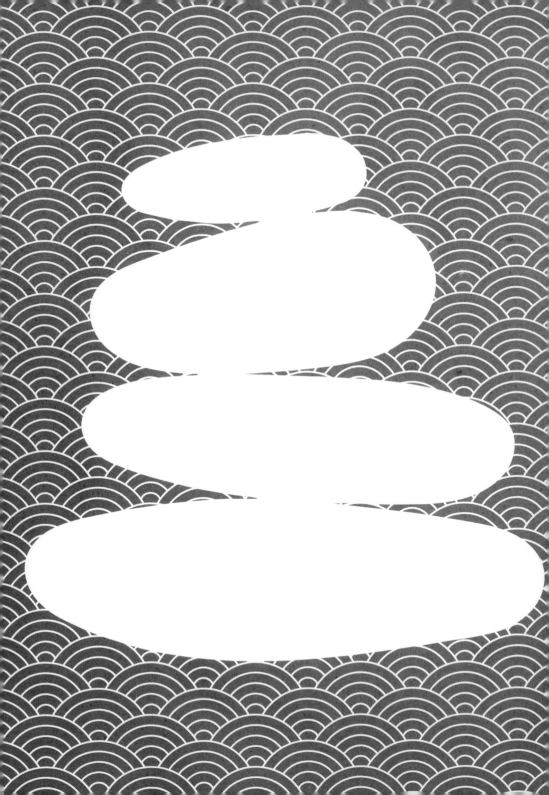

LESSON 15:
BE THOUGHTFUL

Think about a person you feel close to; maybe it's a family member, a friend, or a mentor. Then think about what makes them important to you, and why you both get along so well. What do they do or say differently from other people? How is your relationship different with them than it is with, say, an acquaintance? Most likely, you will describe this person as someone who understands you, or "just gets you" – an act that requires being thoughtful.

I think it is in these moments of understanding that close relationships are born. One of my closest friends today I actually knew for a couple of years before we became good friends. She was funny and kind, and we had several mutual friends, but we had always known each other as classmates. We would sometimes exchange notes to study for an exam, or occasionally sit next to each other during lunch, but our interactions were casual.

This changed one day when I was getting ready for PE. I realized that I had forgotten my gym clothes, and I only had 10 minutes before class started. I began rushing around the locker room to see if there were any lost-and-found items that I could perhaps salvage as a temporary solution. After a heart-racing search, I found a sweaty bright yellow t-shirt and oversized red basketball shorts, but this brought me little relief. I could already imagine how unattractive I'd look in them and the thought of wearing someone else's sweaty t-shirt also made me nauseous.

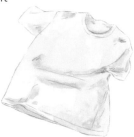

Perhaps it was the frown on my face or my silence that gave it away, but my friend approached me and asked if I was okay.

"Um, yeah, I forgot my gym clothes."

She looked down at the yellow t-shirt and basketball shorts in my hand, and then back at me.

"Oh. I have extra clothes if you'd like them. Sorry, I unfortunately don't have socks though."

She seemed a little surprised by my reaction. I'm not sure I had grinned so hard in front of her before. I profusely thanked her for saving me from having to look like a McDonald's character, and we began giggling at the embarrassing situation saved.

That's when I knew I wanted to be her best friend.

I don't think it'll come as a surprise to many people that building meaningful relationships requires being thoughtful. We grow closer to those who are attentive to our needs, and show consideration toward that which we aren't always comfortable verbally saying. Like being handed a hot coffee on your way out to work, saved from an uncomfortable 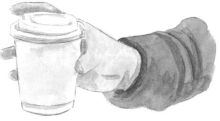 conversation, or being asked what's wrong even if you haven't said anything, we appreciate and grow closer to those who can read what we may need and act on it. In other words, we grow closer to people who understand us.

What many of us may not have paused to think about is how being understood is not something that passively happens, but is one person actively trying to understand the other. It requires being attentive and mindful of someone other than yourself, and while it is often easier to understand someone who is similar to you, we can also learn to be attentive to the needs of people who share different values and perspectives from ourselves when we practice empathy. Being thoughtful doesn't necessitate being empathetic, but when we are able to practice thoughtfulness through empathy, we are able to reach that point where being thoughtful is not just an act of being kind, but something that allows us to understand someone and grow closer with them.

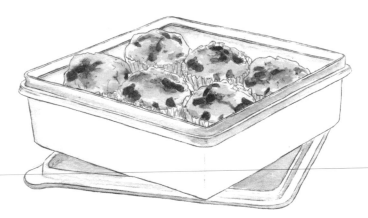

I learned this important lesson when I made the unfortunate mistake of gifting a Japanese person food in Tupperware. One weekend when I had baked a few too many chocolate chip muffins, my mom suggested I give away a few of them to our next-door neighbor. An opportunity to do something nice, I decided to box them up and handed it over that very afternoon. They seemed delighted, and I left feeling happier after my small act.

I was surprised when a few days later, I came home to my mom who had an annoyed look on her face, accusing me, "Why did you give away the muffins in a Tupperware box?"

I stammered and said something about how that was the only clean container we had. I wasn't quite sure what the mistake was, for I thought I was doing something thoughtful. She sighed and shook her head. She explained, you are not to give away food in Tupperware – I thought to myself: what?

In Japan it is considered rude to bring back an empty container, so over time it has become customary for a receiver to bring back some other food when they return Tupperware to the owner, an act known as *okaeshi*. Mindful of this, the extra considerate giver will now be careful to use disposable containers when gifting food, so the receiver isn't burdened with the pressure to give something back. I thought my mother was being ridiculous when she first shared this information with me, that no person thinks like that and they wouldn't feel such pressure. But of course I was proven wrong – a few days later, sitting on our table was our Tupperware box, not empty, but filled with small brownies.

To give away food in a disposable container is to let the other person know that they are welcome to the gift and that they are under no obligation to return the favor. It's an act of thoughtfulness that is not just about being kind, but being attentive to one's needs through empathy. The layered consideration may sometimes feel like a bit too much, but it was at this moment that I realized how lucky I was, for the standard in my community was not only to do good and expect nothing in return, but to also do good and not make the other person feel indebted. It is a value not just shared in my apartment building, but prevalent enough to be considered common sense in Japan.

This is important because however inadvertently, sometimes our good deeds come with a price tag – how often do we silently think, I did the laundry last time, is it now not your turn? – which creates nothing but another's resentment in unsolicited indebtedness and our own frustration when our expectations are not met. But our bitterness will age us, and we lose out on the most valuable thing we have to gain when we approach good deeds quid pro quo.

It might seem like a tedious thing to take consideration of others this far, that gift-giving in Tupperware seems hardly of importance, but it is this underlying sentiment to empathize beyond the surface level that is key to building strong relationships with others. This level of thoughtfulness is how we learn to understand each other, and build a relationship that feels so natural that no dialogue needs to be shared. While sometimes we like to think of someone understanding us as an intuitive and intrinsic connection, in reality, building this understanding takes time and an active effort to empathize with someone else.

There is a Japanese belief, *omoiyari* (思いやり), that is frequently used to describe this empathy for others. It can be understood as the importance of putting yourself in someone else's shoes, but goes one step beyond that – it is not just about emotionally empathizing with someone, but anticipating their needs and meeting them in advance before they need to ask. It's an act that forces us to reflect: What can we do to make someone else's life more pleasant?

While it takes a bit of time to build lasting relationships, we don't need to wait to get closer to people to reap the benefits of thoughtfulness. Our wellbeing already stands to gain when we do good for others. Altruistic behavior and emotions have been shown to be positively correlated with greater happiness and wellbeing.[71] Some studies even show that providing social

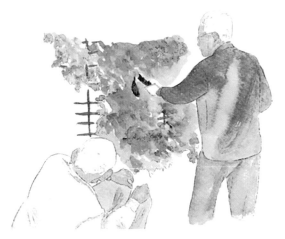

support can help promote longevity[72] and reduce physical pain.[73] In one study, participants who engaged in altruistic behavior experienced lowered blood pressure compared to participants who hadn't,[74] and this decrease in pressure was comparable to what starting exercise or a healthy diet could've done in the same amount of time. Even if our acts of thoughtfulness aren't reciprocated, we only stand to gain from reaching out.

To exemplify, *omoiyari* is to practice *kokorozukai* (心遣い), or using your heart to act for others. It's a practice that is not just unique to Japan, but can be found anywhere you live – inviting someone over to join you for lunch when they're sitting alone, surprising someone with a homemade meal when they're going through a hard time, or even something as small as being mindful of being quiet on the train so as to not disturb other passengers is using your heart to act for others.

Kokorozukai is done with the intention of not just making someone's life easier, but the purpose is to make someone else feel emotionally better. By definition it implies selfless intentions. It is by doing something generous for someone else in a way that would not make them feel indebted that we gain other people's trust. To do otherwise would make our thoughtful deeds become an exchange of goods and services, a context where meaningful relationships can't be born. So instead lead with your heart to do good and then let your good deeds go forgotten, for this is where close relationships are made.

Maybe we don't need to go as far as being sensitive to whether we gift food in Tupperware or not, but the premise is the same – to build meaningful connections with others, we must first embody empathetic thoughtfulness, an act that is not just about practicing kindness but about taking it one step further and truly matching our kindness with the other person's needs and feelings. To grow closer with others is to take the time to understand them: How can we make their life more pleasant?

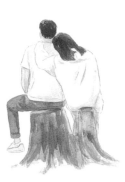

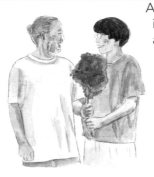

Answering this question implies altruistic intentions, or acting in a way that doesn't allow the other person to feel indebted to generosity. Whether that be to make someone else more cheerful, more comfortable, or more confident, to uplift the spirit of others by leveraging our own ability to empathize is one that allows us to more closely connect with others. While we may hope that they return the gesture with trust and an intention to understand us back, to hold their emotions hostage is not how we break those barriers. Trust is not found in transactions but by practicing empathetic thoughtfulness, and through these acts we will eventually find someone who will want to learn to "just get us" too.

"To grow closer to others is to take the time to understand them."

Lesson 15: Be thoughtful

STRAWBERRY *DAIFUKU*

4 servings

It's always thoughtful to gift your neighbors or friends with desserts, whether you want to thank them for something they did for you or you just want to offer a sweet gesture. Strawberry *daifuku* is relatively easy, quick, vegan, and allergen-free so is the perfect option to share with others. This dessert recipe also doesn't require an oven or any baking, so even if you don't have access to one this is still applicable to you!

Ingredients

- 8 fresh strawberries, stems removed
- 250g/9oz sweet red bean paste
- 110g/3¾oz shiratamako (or sweet rice flour, may be labeled mochiko)
- 40g/1½oz sugar
- 130ml/4¼fl oz/½ cup room temperature water
- potato starch as necessary

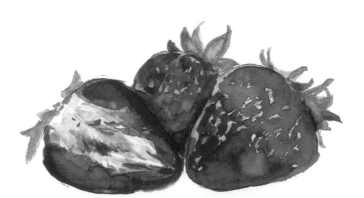

Instructions

1. Clear a large workspace or work on a few large plates. Using your hands, mold the red bean paste into 8 small balls. Using the palm of your hand or a spoon, lightly squash them so they are about ¼ inch flat each.
2. Gently wrap each strawberry in the red bean paste, so it is fully covered.
3. In a glass microwave-safe bowl, add the shiratamako, sugar, and room temperature water. Cover and microwave for 2–2.5 minutes at 600W.
4. Using a rubber spatula, mix together the mochi dough. Cover and microwave for another 1–1.5 minutes at 600W.
5. Using a rubber spatula, mix together the mochi dough again until it is uniform throughout. Set aside.
6. Cover your hands and the workspace with potato starch, and then lay out the mochi dough flat on top so it is about ¼ inch thick. Using a knife, gently cut into 8 pieces. (If the dough cools down too much, it becomes difficult to manipulate, so try to work while it is still warm!)
7. Using your hands mold mochi pieces so they take on a round disc shape. (Make sure your hands and workspace are covered in enough potato starch to prevent sticking.)
8. Gently wrap the sweet bean-strawberry center from earlier with the mochi. Set aside in the fridge for at least 15 minutes so its shape stabilizes.
9. Enjoy!

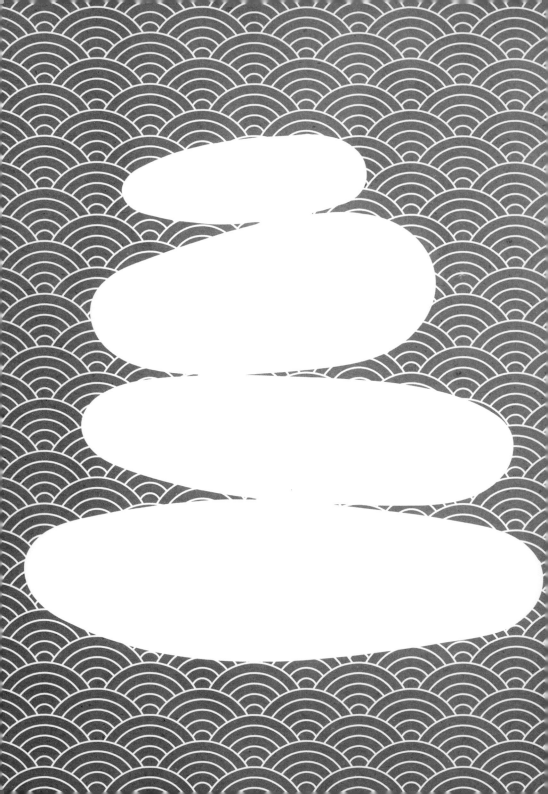

LESSON 16:
SHARE EXPERIENCES

When we meet someone who is interested in getting to know us better, someone who is open and excited about understanding us, sometimes we miss the opportunity to nurture these beginnings. Like all living beings, a relationship is also a living thing that must be cared for and encouraged to grow. While our most valuable relationships end up feeling effortless over time, that stability is the result of time and energy, and in those early green stages of a new relationship, we should be prepared to proactively tend and care for it.

This might sound like a chore, but tending to our relationships is not very complicated, and it should not feel difficult either. This is because we should nurture relationships with not just people we want to spend more time with, but also with people who want to spend more time with us – and if both those measures are met, then being able to make time for and invest in others should become something that we feel excited about and look forward to doing.

It may seem like an obvious answer, but one of the most effective ways to look after a relationship is to share experiences with others.

There is a proverb in Japanese that goes, "Eaten alone, even sea bream does not taste delicious." It may sound strange to someone not familiar with Japanese culture, but sea bream is a highly coveted food and is associated with celebratory occasions in Japan. The proverb means that even the most celebratory occasions don't feel meaningful when we are celebrating alone, and it is the presence of other people and being able to share those happy moments which makes an event significant to us.

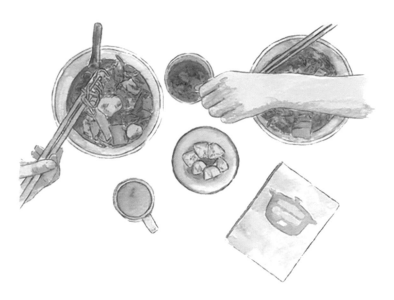

It is not just true as a proverb: food sharing is a powerful way for us to build meaningful relationships and has been shown to support both our physical and mental health. In a meta-analysis published in 2018, researchers found that controlling for children's ages, the country they were from, family structure, or socioeconomic group, there was a significant positive relationship between children who grew up with frequent family meals and better nutritional health.[75] It did not matter if they were rich or poor, grew up in a nuclear family or a single-parent household: if they ate with their family, they were more likely to be healthier later in life. In a similar study published in 2010, researchers went one step further and found that children who grew up with mealtime environments that facilitated family interactions also benefited from better mental health as well.[76] It's not only children who benefit; anybody at any age can benefit from spending more time eating with others. Research published in 2017 suggested that social eating can help individuals feel happier, more satisfied, and engaged with their social circles than those who don't.[77] It wasn't merely a correlation the researchers found, but that social eating practices contributed to psychological benefits, rather than the other way around.

While I provide this evidence, most of us may not need to read a study to understand the influential role of food and mealtimes in our social life. Many of us grow up understanding that food is not just fuel, but also a critical part of how we connect with others. When the holidays come around we celebrate with large meals and decadent cakes, and when we go out to hang out with our friends it often revolves around food and drink. Across countries and generations, it does not necessarily matter where you are from or how old you are, food is often involved in our celebrations, holidays, interests, and simply what we do for fun with others. It's a wonderful way to grow closer with people and nurture our relationships.

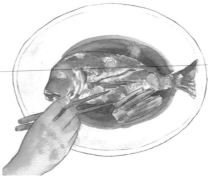

Sharing food is one common way that we learn to share experiences, but sharing experiences doesn't always need to be spending quality time together. While spending time with others is usually the most common and perhaps easiest way, there are other ways we can translate this same intent. One distinctly popular method in Japan is the practice of *omiyage*, or gift giving.

Gift-giving culture is prevalent throughout the world in many different countries, but the practice in Japan is perhaps one of the most extensive. Gift giving in Japan is not only reserved for special occasions such as weddings and birthdays, or as tokens of appreciation and gratitude; it also encompasses the practice of giving for the simple purpose of sharing what one has experienced with another person.

The Japanese word *omiyage* translates to souvenir, but many Japanese people see *omiyage* not as simple souvenir-buying, but as an important part of its relationship-building culture. Unlike western cultures such as in the US or UK, instead of buying mementos for your time in a different country or city, buying souvenirs is largely seen as something you do for other people rather than for yourself.

Omiyage gift giving practices date back centuries in Japan, and were first used when individuals made their way home from long journeys visiting and praying at Shinto shrines. The act of bringing back gifts was used as a way to report to one's family that they had successfully reached their destination and to share with them what they had experienced and learned. Because people could not travel as readily and safely at the time, having just a single family representative go was a way for the family to be a part of that experience even if they could not all physically be there.

Omiyage used to be made up of religious objects, but as traveling became more frequent among the general population, shrines began selling local products to keep up with the rising demand. In this way, *omiyage* eventually changed to be more oriented toward local foods, artisan crafts, and regional goods. Although *omiyage* is no longer just for religious journeys, the sentiment of wanting to share an experience with someone who couldn't be there with you at the time remains today. Whether it be to thank your coworkers who carried the load while you were gone, or your family who were not able to join you on your trip, *omiyage* is used to let others know that even while you were gone, they were on your mind.

Omiyage is not a replacement for quality time with others, but when we can't physically be with the people we are grateful for, it at least gives us an opportunity to talk about what we have seen and heard, and share stories of what we have learned. It shows that we want them to be involved in our lives, and however indirectly, is a simple way of letting someone else in on our memory. Letting others know that they were being thought of in this way can help us create moments of belonging and strengthen our relationships.

I remember when I was very young, my dad went on a business trip to Taiwan for a few days. I was too young to understand why he was leaving at the time, and couldn't help but feel a little neglected. What was my dad doing without me? That could've been the end of the story, but that's not how I remember it now – what I remember is that when he came back, he gave me a bunny-shaped card case made out of pink felt. In handing me the gift, he ended up talking about what he had seen, what he had eaten, how it was different from Japan and the US, and even described the crowded little stall where he bought my gift. Instead of feeling jealous or upset, I was so excited about my little pink bunny card case that I felt happy for him, and glad that he went to Taiwan. It was not the card case I was excited about for I had no cards to really put in it. What made me so happy was that he was thinking about me while he was away, which made his time in Taiwan feel like something we shared.

"Small acts can do a lot to increase our sense of closeness with others, as long as it says to someone else, Hey, I was thinking of you."

It is not the actual object of *omiyage* that matters; it is the intent behind the gift – that the person's presence was missed. Sometimes the gift can be a physical object, but this intent can also be shared through sending photos, text messages, a link to an interesting article we read, or even a funny meme we think someone may enjoy. Small acts can do a lot to increase our sense of closeness with others, as long as it says to someone else, Hey, I was thinking of you.

Sharing experiences with others is important because it builds trust, and when we forget or neglect to involve others in our lives, our relationships can weaken and wane over time. While this is especially true for new relationships where trust and bond are yet to be nurtured, even our most treasured relationships can meet a similar fate if we fail to show that we value their company. We need to make time for and communicate with others that we care about and be invested in maintaining our relationship with them.

Best case scenario, we can spend quality time with the people around us, and physically share those memories with the people we care about. But even if we are limited by time or distance, we can at least fill the interim spaces by reminding them that they are still on our mind and a part of our life. What is not of major importance is what we do or share, but simply letting others know that their presence is welcomed and appreciated.

Lesson 16: Share experiences

JAPANESE *NABEMONO*

4 servings

Nabemono, often known as hot pot in the United States, is a popular wintertime dish in Japan and is arguably one of the most perfect meals you can have. Not only is it incredibly healthy due to its base of vegetables, but it is also an amazingly natural way to bring people together.

Nabemono requires very little preparation and the cooking is done as you eat – so even on your sluggish days when you don't have much time or energy, you can still easily bring it together. Turn on the table-top stove, heat up some dashi in hot water, and cook the food over the pot with some family or friends.

Essential tools
- Portable gas stove
- Big Japanese clay pot

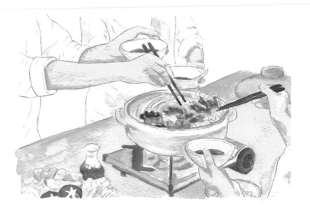

Ingredients
- basic dashi or fish-based kombu broth (I usually buy mine from Kayanoya)
- 400g/14oz thinly sliced pork or beef
- vegetables (washed and cut):
    - napa cabbage
    - leek
    - carrots
    - mushrooms (enoki, shimeji, shiitake)
    - spinach
- other: tofu, mochi rice cakes, or udon noodles

Instructions
1. Place the portable stove on the table, with the clay pot on top. Add the dashi to the pot as instructed and put on high heat.
2. Once it starts simmering, lower the heat and add in cut vegetables, meat, and noodles to personal liking.
3. Enjoy with friends and family!

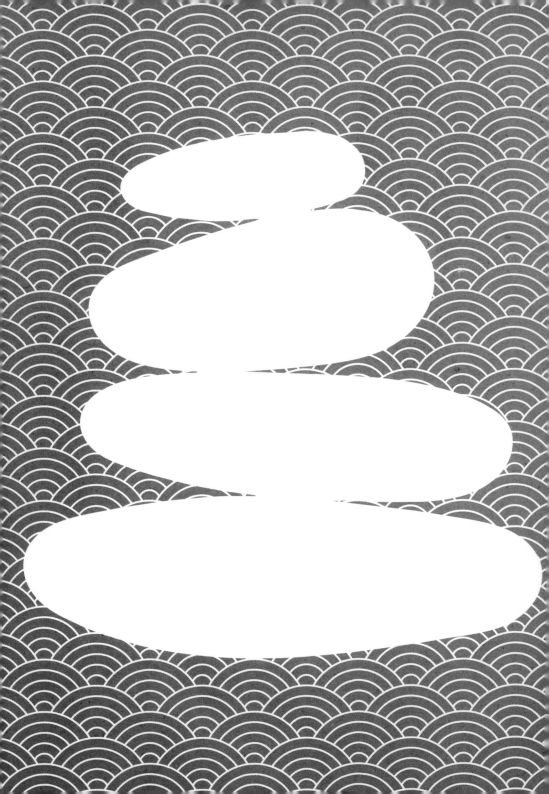

LESSON 17:

QUIET THE EGO

In the art of finding, building, and nurturing our personal relationships into meaningful ones, you may have noticed an underlying principle that runs through all the lessons: instead of focusing on what others can do for us, it's often about how we can serve others with no expectation of anything in return. This does not mean we should have no boundaries or we should invest our energy into those who do not appreciate what we offer, but by placing the focus on the other person rather than ourselves, we build the confidence that the right people will choose us, instead of fearing that there is something about ourselves that needs to change. Paying attention to other people not only benefits others, it also builds our own self-esteem.

Pushing aside one's own ego for others is a valued principle in Japanese society, one that may be most famously demonstrated during the 2018 FIFA World Cup. It was an exciting day for Japanese football fans in June of that year when Japan won its first match against Colombia 2-1. It was the country's first victory against a South American country in the tournament. However, it wasn't the Japanese football team but the Japanese fans in the stadium who made news headlines that day, and for a reason completely unrelated to the outcome of the match – the world was shocked by how meticulously they cleaned their rows and seats when they left the stadium.

Japanese fans had brought their own trash bags and could be seen picking up litter after the match. It was not the first time Japanese fans had been witnessed doing this after a match, but because it was following such a large and historical win, and at a stadium in Russia where that is not a very common custom, many spectators were surprised. Instead of racing off to celebrate and party with other fans, people were staying to clean up – what would entice a group of people to do that? Perhaps because after winning a high stakes match we tend to feel more confident, we also end up feeling more gracious. When we are happy, we tend to be kinder to the people around us and have the emotional bandwidth to be considerate to others as well.

But the following match against Belgium in the same tournament resulted in a devastating loss for Japan. Japan was winning 2-0 but ended up being beaten 2-3 with only 25 minutes left on the clock. After losing a much-anticipated game, you would think that the fans would be upset, frustrated, or even angry, and that cleaning up the stadium would be the last thing on their mind. However, putting aside any personal feelings, many people still came together to leave the stadium as clean as they had found it. Win or lose, fans stayed after the game to pick up after themselves.

"By seeing yourself as a part of something much grander than what lives in your own mind, you can find emotional freedom."

How did the Japanese fans and players feel after this match? It would be reasonable to feel dejected after a loss, but surprisingly, cleaning up after the game had made many people leave the stadium with a much different emotion. Instead of being upset, many fans and players felt that the loss was overshadowed by how proud and grateful they were that they could finish the tournament with dignity and respect to their hosts.[78] They were upset about the loss of course, but by being conscious of the bigger purpose behind the World Cup tournament, many of them were able to emotionally rise above it.

Pride is hardly a feeling that one might expect after such a surprising loss, but by shifting our focus, we can shape the narrative of how we are supposed to feel. This is just one example of how putting aside our self-importance – or our ego – can help us regain our confidence and become less manipulated by our negative emotions. It is not necessarily about making yourself smaller, but by seeing yourself as a part of something much grander than what lives in your own mind, you can find emotional freedom and control through the larger perspective.

While American culture often champions the individual and the uniqueness each person brings, Japanese culture often moves in the opposite direction, where its values lie in a person's ability to contribute to the larger community. Rather than a desire to be special or outstanding, many people are taught to seek being useful, collaborative, or someone that others can rely on. Americans can be quick to point out the flaws of a collectivist culture – I understand and agree that there are drawbacks as well – but there are priceless advantages to being a part of a society that champions the greater whole over the individual. For myself, there have been two specific times in my life where I have felt extreme gratitude and indebtedness to this quieting of the ego.

The first was when I was in Japan during the March 11th Fukushima disaster in 2011. I remember that day like an American remembers 9/11. I was in school and there were only a few minutes on the clock until my last class ended, when the entire building began to shake. Earthquakes are quite common in Japan and so at first no one took it too seriously, slowly lumbering to get under the too-small desks, but it suddenly became strong and violent. Even once the first quake had stopped, teachers looked worried and everyone was confused.

I pulled out my phone in an attempt to contact my family or check the news, but with everyone in the country trying to do the same, cellular and Internet connection quickly shut down and it was impossible to reach anyone. Getting home from school usually only took about half an hour, but that day I remember sitting on the bus for over six hours due to traffic and congestion. The city was in chaos.

It was only when I was finally able to reunite with my family at home and watch the news that I finally understood the gravity of what had happened. News of a powerful earthquake, a ferocious tsunami which swept up a city, and a nuclear power plant meltdown were running headlines on the screen. My life in Japan had always been very safe and comfortable for me, but suddenly all my beliefs around stability were uprooted and questioned. School was temporarily canceled, many of my friends left Japan, and I wasn't supposed to leave the house for fear of radiation poisoning. There was so much paranoia and fear in the air.

You might expect that with this much fear, some people may have tried to take advantage of this crisis. It is not unheard of for people to start looting, to vandalize, or for other crimes to go up. Sometimes people try to surge-price necessary goods like water or toilet paper, and some may try to bulk buy these items, meaning others may not be able to access them. In times of crisis, it's very common for people to only think about their own needs; it's almost understandable. So I was very surprised when after 3/11, the widespread violence I expected never materialized – there were cases here and there, but on the whole there was no looting, no drastic increases in crime and no havoc. In fact, for several weeks Tokyo was very quiet and sullen.

This was the first time I learned of the term *jishuku* (自粛). *Jishuku* is loosely defined as the practice of restraining from luxury and celebration in consideration of others who are going through a difficult time. Then-Prime Minister Abe encouraged citizens to practice *jishuku*, to show support for those directly affected by the disasters. *Jishuku* was not just for the victims, but for the volunteers and workers who were going out of their way to rebuild homes and clean up radioactive waste as well. The idea was that those who couldn't directly help should at least show support by restraining themselves from going out, and to patiently wait until the dust settled down for everyone.

Springtime is one of the most celebrated seasons in Japan, for it is when students graduate from school, fresh-grads begin to start new jobs, and when cherry blossom festivals and events are hosted to welcome back the warmer weather. Spring is typically associated with joy and fun, but that year many of these major events were canceled or postponed. It was not forever, and eventually society reopened and business went back to normal, but I'll always remember how on a national level, so many people came together for a moment to show support. There was fear and uncertainty, but it didn't turn Japanese society against each other – the wealthy did not host lavish parties, and the reckless did not go on looting sprees to capitalize on others' misfortune. On the whole, people were staying at home and keeping quiet in consideration of others.

Experiences of disaster – in particular, the resulting housing damage and loss – have been associated with increased risk of

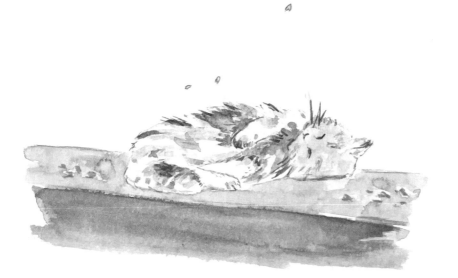

mental illness in people,[79] but a study published in 2017 found that our social connections can help buffer that association.[80] Of those who had lost their homes in the earthquake and tsunami disaster in 2011, individuals who lived in communities with strong social networks were less likely to suffer from dementia later on in life compared to those who did not have as many opportunities for social participation in their communities. Even casual and apparently mundane socializing such as visiting a neighbor was found to mitigate the risk of dementia. Supporting and feeling supported is critical for people's health.

"When we quiet the ego and place priority on the wellbeing of the group over the individual, we all stand to benefit."

The second time I felt grateful for Japan's collectivist values was when the coronavirus pandemic emerged in 2020. It felt very similar to when the 2011 earthquake happened: how schools closed, graduation ceremonies were canceled, annual festivities were shut down, and most people ended up spending their spring vacations at home. This time around, the willingness for individuals to adhere to these actions was even more critical, for *jishuku* was directly about preventing the spread of the virus to protect the lives of the immunocompromised and at-risk. It was not necessarily fun or convenient, but like in 2011, people dutifully obliged.

And it was worthwhile. As of writing in May of 2022, Japan's coronavirus deaths per million stands at 233.19. For comparison, the US stands at 2,995.28 per million and the UK at 2,574.71 per million.[81] This isn't meant to be an evaluation of countries or cultures, but what I've seen in Japan has proven to me that a successful coronavirus containment doesn't mean having to give up personal freedom or liberty: there was no forced government lockdown or threatening fines for breaking social distancing rules, and Japanese citizens were allowed to continue to choose how they'd like to live their day to day. Stay at home or go out? Wear a mask or leave it at home?

When we quiet the ego and place priority on the wellbeing of the group over the individual, we all stand to benefit. Being able to see our role in the larger picture and the influence we have on the wellbeing of others allows us to build meaningful connections with our community, which in return will protect and serve our health as well. While I love and appreciate the sense of individualism and value of self-expression my upbringing in the US has shown me, self-importance is not the only way we can learn to carry pride and confidence in ourselves. Sometimes focusing on what we can do for others is what increases our sense of wellbeing.

Quieting the ego may not always feel like an easy task, for our ego is an instinctual form of survival, but being able to disengage with our self-importance can bring us joy and improve our lives. We do not need to complicate or be intimidated by the endeavor; all we must do to learn is start with the question: What influence do I have on the community around me right now? From there we can find small acts of how we may be able to benefit and help others – picking up after ourselves, checking on our neighbor, or sometimes simply staying at home can do a world of good for everyone.

Lesson 17: Quiet the ego

CONCLUSION:
WHAT *WA* LOOKS LIKE IN REAL LIFE

I have a confession: my life is not the perfect vision of an optimal healthy life. I sometimes sleep a little too late, or find myself eating ice cream a few too many nights in a row. You will catch me forgetting to stretch after a long day sitting down at a desk, and sometimes I will go the entire day without leaving the house. I sometimes eat too much meat, and can be found staring and scrolling through my phone on the couch for too long.

But having room for these "unhealthy" habits is precisely why I can lead a healthy life. To not give myself permission to engage with them is to treat myself like a computer, rather than a person.

Let's take a moment to reflect on and visualize what it means to you to live healthfully. What would your life look like? What would you be spending your time doing and thinking about? For most of us, we would like the healthiest version of ourselves to not be overly concerned with details like counting macros, tracking calories burned, or otherwise being stressed or worried by the prospect of our health. We would want our bodies to be physically fit and strong, but also our minds to be sound and at peace. We would want contentment and to feel emboldened, rather than limited, by our bodies and minds.

When we think about health in this way, we quickly realize that good health is not just about being concerned with eating vegetables or working out regularly, or sleeping at a reasonable hour and spending time in nature. At the higher level, it's about paying attention to our health so that we can explore the

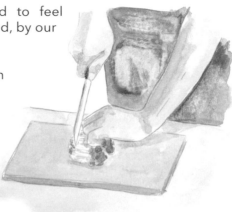

world in ways that are most meaningful to us. We want to enjoy quality time with our loved ones, and travel to learn more about different cultures and ways of living. We want to explore and go on adventures without being held back by our health, and have the energy to be curious about the things that interest us. We want to eat good food and share drinks with close friends. But to do these things, we need to realize that sometimes we must be comfortable doing the "unhealthy" thing as well: to occasionally enjoy desserts, eat fried foods, sleep late, or skip going on a run. Good health is about freedom and possibility, not restriction or rules – and the key to achieving this is understanding the art of balance.

A healthy life is a seemingly simple idea, but it can be difficult to vocalize and describe. While the traditional narrative is one that is focused on exercise and diet, it is helpful to expand our scope to the mind and pay attention to our wellbeing as something holistic. Our physical and mental health are closely interrelated, and to not recognize and hold empathy for our humanness is an approach that tends to be unsustainable over the course of our lifetime. Instead, when we put our quality of life first – and hold space to be a little mindful of balance – then we can trust that everything else about our health will follow.

Working out every day for hours and putting yourself on a restrictive diet will get you results faster – but it can also lead to burnout, stress, and frustration much quicker too. It might get us to our physical markers, but what good is a number on a scale or diagram if it can never give us contentment and peace? Whenever you feel lost on your health journey, think back to your optimal healthy life – are the actions you are taking conducive to that vision?

> "Good health is about freedom and possibility, not restriction and rules and the key to achieving this is understanding the art of balance."

Embarking and embodying a *wa* approach to health is not one that may feel like your typical health journey. It rarely feels pivotal in one's life, and may come off as a more subtle undercurrent behind our typical daily decisions.

In terms of nourishment, it might just be setting aside your dinner plate a little earlier than usual and saving the rest to take home. It might be adding a serving of herbs to your pasta rather than topping it off with more cheese for flavor. It might be nudging your idea of decadence from one rooted in caloric value, to one that is focused on quality and artisanal care.

With movement, it might be about choosing to do a short yoga routine after a long day of sitting at work, or choosing to take the train to work rather than a car. It might mean going outside for a jog instead of going back to the treadmill. It can even be about paying less attention to calories burned, and more attention to how joyful you find the exercise itself.

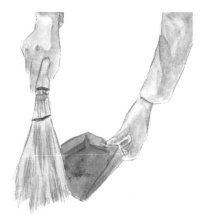

With rest, it may be about occasionally setting aside enough time to enjoy cooking, rather than always pushing yourself to be as efficient as possible in the kitchen. It might be about spending that extra time to notice details about the ingredients, and allowing yourself the bandwidth to experiment and be curious about food. Or maybe it's just about spending a few seconds making the bed in the morning so at night you are welcomed to a clean, tidy bed. It can be about taking on the mindset of curiosity to slow down and allow yourself a bit of time to breathe and relax.

With socializing, it can be smiling and saying hello before you order a drink at your local coffee shop. It might be buying a dinosaur book in the museum bookshop for your co-worker's dinophile child or holding the door open for someone with their hands full. It can even be as simple as being mindful of your volume on the subway car when you notice there's a baby sleeping next to you.

"To approach our health with a balanced mindset is to be empathetic of our humanness."

These are subtle changes, but compounded over the course of our lifetime, they have the potential to redirect our health in very powerful ways. The kind gesture can increase our sense of confidence, and maybe nudge us to try a more challenging workout. That workout can allow us to find better sleep at night, and in turn we may find ourselves eating healthier because we feel less stressed. The four pillars, and the mental and physical health considerations embedded in them, are all very closely interrelated in ways that are both obvious and not so obvious to us. But strengthen one pillar, and we lift others as well.

To approach our health with a balanced mindset is to be empathetic of our humanness, and the details that make ourselves and our lives unique. Instead of seeing choices as right or wrong, or to take on one extreme over another, enjoy the process of finding your unique middle ground and what works for you. This acknowledgement of our humanness is what allows us to lean into the experimentation process and find sustainability in the journey, rather than be overwhelmed or become guilt-ridden by our choices. When we embrace the art of balance in this way, we learn an approach toward health that allows us to live healthier, happier, and longer lives.

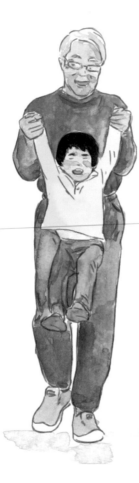

ABOUT THE AUTHOR

Sakiko Ohashi (pen name: Kaki Okumura) is a certified nutritional therapy practitioner and writes on Japanese food, fitness, lifestyle, and health. Her writing on *Medium* garners hundreds of thousands of views a month, and she has also been featured in *Bon Appetit*, *Eater*, *Heated x Mark Bittman*, and Katie Couric's newsletter *Wake Up Call*. She occasionally speaks on podcasts, interviews professional chefs, and posts cooking videos. She likes to create beautiful illustrations for everything.

Follow her on Instagram @kakikata.space or join her highly regarded newsletter at www.kakikata.space. If you really like her writing, send her an email (it's shared when you join the newsletter) – she loves to read everything that comes her way.

ACKNOWLEDGMENTS

How does one begin to thank everyone who has helped write this book? Whenever I took the time to read the acknowledgements in the books I've read, it always astounded me the number of names that popped up. I now understand why.

I'd first like to thank my parents and sisters for unconditionally supporting me, even before I knew what I was doing myself. From looking over my drafts and steering me back on track when I was getting distracted, to making sure I was eating when I was holed up in my room typing away. It is inevitable for there to be both celebratory and hard moments in lifen - I feel grateful that I can share both the ups and downs with you guys.

I'd also like to thank my agent Michele, for opening that door and asking, "Hey, have you ever considered writing a book?" I wouldn't have expected it at the time, but wow, it has ended up somewhere wonderful.

Finally, a big thank you to the entire Watkins team. I'm no expert in publishing, marketing, or book design, so I feel so lucky to have such a talented team to back my writing and make this possible. A special thank you to editors Ella and Brittany for believing in the book and for doing the hard part of taking a vision and transforming it into reality. I'm very grateful for your patience. And thank you to Hayley, for taking a jumble of ideas and words into something that readers can enjoy. The talent of others will never cease to amaze me.

ENDNOTES

1. company.bk.com/pdfs/nutrition.pdf

2. www.worldometers.info/demographics/life-expectancy/

3. obesity.procon.org/global-obesity-levels/

4. www.helgilibrary.com/indicators/rice-consumption-per-capita/ japan/

5. Kawasaki, Tamaki, "Meiji and the Dawn of Modern Civilization in Japan", *Highlighting Japan*, vol.125, October 2018, pp6-7

6. Jubala, Jullian, "9 Impressive Health benefits of cabbage", *Healthline*, 4 November 2017

7. Patel, A D et al, "Review on Biochemical Importance of Vitamin-U. J", *Chem. Pharm. Res.*, 4(1), 2012, pp209-215

8. www.bluezones.com/about/history/

9. Alam M A et al, "Beneficial Role of Bitter Melon Supplementation in Obesity and Related Complications in Metabolic Syndrome", *J Lipids*, 2015

10. Willcos, Craig et al, "Aging Gracefully: a Retrosective Analysis of Functional Status in Okinawan centenarians", *Am J Geriatr Psychiatry*, 15(3), March 2007, pp252-6

11. Ogura, C et al, "Prevalence of Senile Dementia in Okinawa, Japan", *International Journal of Epidemiology*, 24(2), 1995, pp373-80

12. Willcox, Donald Craig et al, "Healthy Aging Diets Other Than the Mediterranean: A Focus on the Okinawan Diet", Mechanisms of Ageing and Development, Vol.136-7, March–April 2014, pp148-162

13. Petre, Alina, "What is Tofu, and Is It Healthy?", *Heathline*, updated 2 February 2022

14. Perry, Charles, "Rot of Ages", *Los Angeles Times*, April 1998

15. yorozu-do.com/work-ranking/#2021

16. Minna no Rankingu, HANABISHI Inc, based on 212 participants, November 2022, net/rankings/best-luxury-foods

17. "Physical Activity", *Centers for Disease Control and Prevention*, www.cdc.gov/physicalactivity/basics/adults/index.htm

18. "Research on Sports and Daily Sports", *Rakuten Insight inc*, based

on 1,000 samples, July 18 to July 19 2018, insight.rakuten.co.jp/
report/20180829/

19. National Health and Nutrition Survey conducted by the Ministry
of Health, Labor, and Welfare, 2019

20. Spitzer, Kirk, "Secrets From the Longest-Living Place on Earth",
AARP, May 2014

21. Ministry of Land, Infrastructure, Transport and Tourism, 2005 Census
(conducted), March 2007 (published), www.mlit.go.jp/kisha/
kisha07/01/010330_3/01.pdf

22. makkoho.or.jp/shiru__history

23. "The Importance of Stretching", *Harvard Health Publishing*, 14 March
2022

24. Malanga, Gerard, "Sitting Diseas and Its Impact on your Spine",
Spine Universe, 14 March 2019

25. "Adding variety to an Exercise Routine Helps Increase Adherence",
University of Florida News, 24 October 2000

26. Susan K Malone et al, "Habitual Physical Activity Patterns in a
Nationally Representative Sample of U.S. Adults", *Translational
Behavioral Medicine*, 11(2), February 2021, pp332–341

27. Jackson, Erica M, "Stress Relief: The Role of Exercise in Stress
Management", *ACSM's Health & Fitness Journal*, 17(3), May–June
2013, pp14–19

28. Park B J et al, "The physiological effects of Shinrin-yoku (taking in
the forest atmosphere or forest bathing): evidence from field
experiments in 24 forests across Japan", *Environ Health Prev
Med*,15(1), January 2010, pp18–26

29. Li, Qing, *Forest Bathing: How Trees Can Help You Find Health and
Happiness*, Viking, April 2018

30. Li Q et al, "A Forest Bathing Trip Increases Human Natural Killer
Activity and Expression of Anti-Cancer Proteins in Female
Subjects", *J Biol Regul Homeost Agents*, 22(1), January–March
2008, pp45–55

31. "Improving Health and Wellness Through Access to Nature", *APHA*,
www.apha.org/policies-and-advocacy/public-health-policy-
statements/policy-database/2014/07/08/09/18/improving-health-
and-wellness-through-access-to-nature

32. "Spenging More Time in Nature Can Improve Young People's
Confidence", *UCL*, November 2019

33. White, MP et al, "Spending at Least 120 Minutes a Week in Nature is Associated with Good Health and Wellbeing", *Sci Rep 9*, 77(30), 2019

34. Stibich, March, "Longevity of Okinawans and Healthy Aging in Blue Zones", *Very Well Health*, April 2020,

35. Goss, Rob, "The Island Unlocked the Secret to Long Life – and Knows How to Get Through Tough Tims", *National Geographic*, October 2020

36. Greer S M, Goldstein A N, Walker M P, "The Impact of Sleep Deprivation on Food Desire in the Human Brain", *Nat Commun*, 4(2259), 2013

37. Babson K A et al, "A Test of the Effects of Acute Sleep Deprivation on General and Specific Self-Reported Anxiety and Depressive Symptoms: An Experimental Extension", *J Behav Ther Exp Psychiatry*, 41(3),. September 2010, pp297–303

38. Bhaskar S, Hemavathy D, Prasad S, "Prevalence of Chronic Insomnia in Adult Patients and its Correlation with Medical Comorbidities", *J Family Med Prim Care*, 5(4), October–December 2016, pp780–784

39. "The Wellbeing Report from Aviva", *Aviva,* based on 2235 respondents, September 2017 (conducted), December 2017 (published)

40. Yanes, Ariana, "Just Say Yes? The Rise of 'Study Drugs' in College", *CNN Health*, April 2014

41. Schwarz, Alan, "Workers Seeking Productivity in a Pill Are Abusing A.D.H.D. Drugs", *New York Times*, April 2015

42. Ruiz, Don Miguel, *The Four Agreements: A Practical guide to Personal Freedom*, Amber-Allen Publishing, 2018

43. Raypole, Crystal, "Hurry Sickness is a Think – Here's Why You Might Want to Slow Down", *Healthline*, January 2021

44. Sõetsu, Yanagi, *The Unknown Craftsman*, Kodansha America, 2013

45. Gotink R A et al, "8-week Mindfulness Based Stress Reduction Induces Brain Changes Similar to Traditional Long-Term Meditation Practice - A Systematic Review", *Brain Cogn*, 108, October 2016, pp32–41

46. Hofmann S G and Gómez A F, "Mindfulness-Based Interventions for Anxiety and Depression", *Psychiatr Clin North Am*, 40(4), December 2016, pp739–749

47. Hughes J W et al, "Randomized Controlled Trial of Mindfulness-Based Stress Reduction for Prehypertension", *Psychosom Med*, 75(8), October 2013, pp721–8

48. McMains S and Kastner S, "Interactions of Top-Down and Bottom-Up Mechanisms in Human Visual Cortex", *J Neurosci*, 31(2), January 2011, pp587–97

49. Gaspar, J M et al, "Inability to Suppress Salient Distractors Predicts Low Visual Working Memory Capacity", *PNAS,* 113(13), February 2016

50. Vartanian L R et al, "Clutter, Chaos, and Overconsumption: The Role of Mind-Set in Stressful and Chaotic Food Environments", *Environment and Behaviour*, 49(2), February 2016

51. www.nippon.com/ja/features/h00226/

52. www.britain-visitor.com/churches-uk

53. Niwano Peace Foundation, study based on 1203 responses, June 2019, www.npf.or.jp/pdf/2019_research.pdf

54. The Institute of Statistical Mathematics, study based on 3170 responses, October –December 2013

55. Blazer, D, "Religion/Spirituality and Depression: What Can We Learn From Empirical Studies?", *The American Journal of Psychiatry*, 169(1), January 2012, pp10-12

56. Dew R E et al, "Religion/Spirituality and Adolescent Psychiatric Symptoms: A Review", *Child Psychiatry Hum Dev*, 39(4), December 2008, pp381–98

57. Schnitker, S A and Emmons, R A, "Patience as a virtue: Religious and Psychological Perspectives", In Research in the *Social Scientific Study of Religion*, Vol.18, 2007, Leiden, The Netherlands: Brill,

58. Schnitker, Sarah A, "An Examination of Patience and Well-Being", *The Journal of Positive Psychology*, 7(4), 2012, pp263–280

59. Saltz, Gail, "Is Gratitude Good for Your Mental Health?", *Health Matters*, healthmatters.nyp.org/is-gratitude-good-for-your-health/.

60. Kavedzija I, "An Attitude of Gratitude: Older Japanese in the Hopeful Present", *Anthropology & Aging*, 41(2), 2020

61. Waldinger, Robert, "What Makes a Good Life? Lessons From the Longest Study on happiness", *TedTalk*

62. Holt-Lunstad J et al, "Loneliness and Social Isolation as Risk Factors for Mortality: A Meta-Analytic Review", *Perspectives on Psychological Science*, 10(2), 2015, pp227–237

63. "Chart 1-2-34", Annual Report on the Ageing Society, Cabinet Office, Government of Japan, Ministry of Health, Labour and Welfare, 2016

64. Saito T et al, "Influence of Social Relationship Domains and Their Combinations on Incident Dementia: a Prospective Cohort Study", *J Epidemiol Community Health*, 72(1), January 2018, pp7–12

65. Lambert N M et al, "Benefits of Expressing Gratitude: Expressing Gratitude to a Partner Changes One's View of the Relationship", *Psychological Science*, 21(4), 2010, pp574–580

66. Waldinger, Robert, "What Makes a Good Life? Lessons From the Longest Study on happiness", *TedTalk*

67. Buecker S et al, "Is Loneliness in Emerging Adults Increasing Over Time? A Preregistered Cross-Temporal Meta-Analysis and Systematic Review", *Psychological Bulletin*, 147(8), 2021, pp787–805

68. Weissbourd, Richard et al, "Loneliness in America: How the Pandemic Has Deepened an Epidemic of Loneliness and What We Can Do About It", *Harvard Graduate School of Education*, February 2021

69. Granovetter, Mark S, "The Strength of Weak Ties", *American Journal of Sociology*, 78(6), 1973, pp1360–80

70. Sandstrom G M and Dunn E W, "Social Interactions and Well-Being: The Surprising Power of Weak Ties", *Personality and Social Psychology Bulletin*, 40(7), 2014, pp910–922

71. Post S G, "Altuism, Happiness, and Health: It's Good to be Good", *Int J Behav Med*, 12(2), 2015, pp66–77

72. Brown S L et al, "Providing Social Support May Be More Beneficial Than Receiving It: Results From a Prospective Study of Mortality", *Psychological Science*, 14(4) 2003, pp320–327

73. Wang Y et al, "Altruistic Behaviors Relieve Physical Pain", *PNAS*, 117(2), December 2019

74. Whillans AV et al, "Is Spending Money on Others Good for Your Heart?", *Health Psychol*, 35(6), June 2016, pp574–83,

75. Dallacker M, Hertwig R and Mata J, "The Frequency of Family Meals and Nutritional Health in Children: A Meta-Analysis", *Obes Rev*, 19(5), May 2018, pp638–653

76. Maynard M J and Harding S, "Ethnic Differences in Psychological Well-Being in Adolescence in the Context of Time Spent in Family

Activities", *Soc Psychiatry Psychiatr Epidemiol*, 45(1), January 2010, pp115–23

77. Dunbar R I M, "Breaking Bread: The Functions of Social Eating", *Adaptive Human Behavior and Physiology,* 3, 2017, pp198–211

78. Johnson, Jesse, "Samurai Blue and Fans Win Praise for Clean Exit, and Dignity in Defeat", *The Japan Times*, July 2018

79. Hikichi H et al, "Increased Risk of Dementia in the Aftermath of the 2011 Great East Japan Earthquake and Tsunami," *PNAS*, 113(45), October 2016

80. Hikichi H et al, "Social Capital and Cognitive Decline in the Aftermath of a Natural Disaster: A Natural Experiment from the 2011 Great East Japan Earthquake and Tsunami", *The Lancet*, 1(3), June 2017

81. www.statista.com/statistics/1104709/coronavirus-deaths-worldwide-per-million-inhabitants

GLOSSARY

aisatsu – greetings

aizuchi – verbal and non-verbal cues during a conversation that indicate to the speaker that the listener is paying attention

arigatō – thank you (casual)

arigatō gozaimasu – thank you (formal, or when you want to express deep gratitude)

aonori – type of seaweed, often dried and powdered

butsudan – a small Buddhist altar

chanpurū – an Okinawan stir-fried vegetable dish

chourei – a morning greeting, often used by Japanese schools and sometimes workplaces

daifuku – Japanese confectionery made of mochi stuffed with a sweet filling, often sweet red bean paste

ganbaru – the idea of putting your best foot forward, or to do your best

gochisousama deshita – a common expression of gratitude after a meal

goma-dofu – tofu-like dish made from ground sesame seeds

harahachi-bunme – the idea that we don't need to be eating until we are full; only until we are satisfied (direct translation: "80 per cent your stomach")

harahachi-bunme, isha irazu – a common Japanese proverb, "Eat in moderation, and you will never need to see another doctor"

GLOSSARY

hayashi rice – a western-style beef stew dish popular in Japan

hijiki – a type of brown sea vegetable

hikikomori – young people who become recluses in their parents' home and refuse to leave their room for months or years at a time

hōjicha – roasted green tea, appears light brown when brewed

hoshii – dehydrated boiled rice

ichiju-sansai – one soup, three sides

irasshaimase – a common polite greeting to welcome someone into a shop, restaurant, or other establishment

irichī – an Okinawan stir-fry

itadakimasu – a common expression of gratitude before a meal

ittekimasu – a common phrase when leaving home or the office, to express you'll be going now but coming back later

jishuku – the practice of restraining from luxury and celebration in consideration of others who are going through a difficult time

jiyu-honpou – a short Japanese proverb that highlights the importance of being able to live in a way that is not bound by the rules and customs of the world, but one that is informed by your own needs and desires

jūshī – an Okinawan rice dish, where vegetables and seasonings are cooked with the rice

Kaki-chan – "chan" is a term of endearment added to the end of someone's name, often babies, young children, young women, or pets

kiku – to listen

kodawari – the relentless pursuit of perfection

GLOSSARY

kokoro – soul or heart

kokorozukai – the act of using your heart for others

kombu – a type of sea vegetable, often used in Japanese broths and seasonings

Makko Ho – a stretching system developed by a Japanese man named Wataru Nagai

mata yoroshiku onegaishimasu – a polite and formal expression to close a conversation, or to express that you look forward to a continued amicable relationship

nabemono – a Japanese hot pot

naruhodo – "I see", a way of confirming you're listening when someone else is speaking

niku-jaga – Japanese meat and potato stew

ohayo – good morning (casual)

ohayo gozaimasu – good morning (formal)

okaeri nasai – welcome home

okaeshi – to return a favor or gift

okura natto – a dish of fermented soybean and lightly boiled okra mixed together

omoiyari – the act of putting yourself in someone else's shoes (empathy)

omiyage – a souvenir bought for someone else

osekihan – rice with Azuki beans

osewa ni narimasu – a polite and formal expression to thank someone for their kindness, support, or hard work osonae – a food offering

Rajio taiso – a short Japanese morning exercise routine, popularized with national radio broadcasts ("rajio" means radio)

sado – the ceremonial preparation and presentation of tea

sansho – a type of pepper

shichimi – seven tastes (staple Japanese seasoning blend)

shinrin-yoku – forest bathing

shokunin – an artisan

shojin-ryori – the traditional dining style of Buddhist monks in Japan

tako-san – "tako" means octopus and "san" is usually a title of respect added to the end of someone's name, but when used for inanimate objects or animals, the personification is used to make it cuter for younger audiences

tamagoyaki – a Japanese sweet, rolled omelette

tang ping – a popular social protest by young Chinese people that describes rejecting marriage, having kids and getting a job, and instead participating in society as little as physically possible

teishoku – Japanese set meal

tsukemono – Japanese pickles, can refer to many different kinds and types

umami – one of the five core tastes (among sweet, salty, bitter, and sour), often described as savoriness

undoukai – sports day

wa – harmony, but is also used to describe Japanese things and ideas

GLOSSARY

wafū hambāgu – a Japanese Hamburg dish

wafuku – Japanese traditional clothing

wagashi – Japanese confectionary

wakame – a type of seaweed, often added to Japanese soups and salads

washi – Japanese paper

washoku – Japanese food

warabi-mochi – a mochi-like Japanese confectionery covered in roasted soybean powder, made from starch rather than glutinous rice

zabuton – a Japanese sitting cushion

zafu – a Japanese traditional meditation cushion

zakkokumai – rice with seeds and grains

INDEX

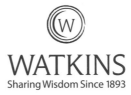

WATKINS

Sharing Wisdom Since 1893

The story of Watkins began in 1893, when scholar of esotericism John Watkins founded our bookshop, inspired by the lament of his friend and teacher Madame Blavatsky that there was nowhere in London to buy books on mysticism, occultism or metaphysics. That moment marked the birth of Watkins, soon to become the publisher of many of the leading lights of spiritual literature, including Carl Jung, Rudolf Steiner, Alice Bailey and Chögyam Trungpa.

Today, the passion at Watkins Publishing for vigorous questioning is still resolute. Our stimulating and groundbreaking list ranges from ancient traditions and complementary medicine to the latest ideas about personal development, holistic wellbeing and consciousness exploration. We remain at the cutting edge, committed to publishing books that change lives.

DISCOVER MORE AT:
www.watkinspublishing.com

Read our blog   Watch and listen to   Sign up to
                    our authors in action   our mailing list

We celebrate conscious, passionate, wise and happy living.
Be part of that community by visiting

  /watkinspublishing   @watkinswisdom
  /watkinsbooks   @watkinswisdom